ANCIENT
SECRETS OF
FACIAL
REJUVENATION

ANCIENT
SECRETS OF
FACIAL
REJUVENATION

a holistic, nonsurgical
approach to youth & well-being

VICTORIA J. MOGILNER, C.A.

NEW WORLD LIBRARY
NOVATO, CALIFORNIA

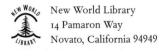
New World Library
14 Pamaron Way
Novato, California 94949

Photographs by David Nanney
Text design and typography by Tona Pearce Myers

ISBN-13: 978-1-57731-552-0

Printed in the U.S.A.

To Auntie Poepoe and Papa Kei,
for teaching the Hawaiian tradition
that love permeates everything we do.

To Dr. Jack Worsely,
for showing me how to live my life in tune with the seasons.

To Betty Mehling, Bonnie Pendleton,
and May Brewmeister,
for knowing the traditions of Jin Shin Jytsu
and for living life with love, truth, and beauty.

There is a star that comes from heaven above to bless the beauty of every woman on Earth. With this gift, there is love, hope, and everlasting travel through the Earth's lifetime. It is a gift of unconditional love for humankind.

— Auntie Mahilani Poepoe

Contents

Chapter Two.
Toward a More Youthful Face ❧ 11

Chapter Three.
Setting the Stage for the Acupressure Facelift ❧ 23

Chapter Four.
The Acupressure Facelift: A Step-by-Step Practice ❦ 33

Chapter Five.
Acupressure Treatments for Common Maladies
That Show in the Face ❦ 63

Chapter Six.
Nutrition for Healthy Skin and a Healthy Body   87

Chapter Seven.
Living in Harmony with the Seasons   107

Chapter Eight.
The Magic of Essential Oils ❧ 125

Chapter Nine.
Your Healthy New Lifestyle ❧ 141

Foreword

There is a soft, sweet, gentle love within our souls and hearts that we rarely acknowledge and even less often embrace. This loving part within each of us is the touchstone at the heart of our Creator. This essence within is a lighted, loving core that feeds us life-force energy, filling us with enthusiasm for all that life sends our way.

Energy surrounds us and affects our every breathing moment, yet we don't often consciously work with it to create an inner balance of emotional and mental peace and exuberant physical health. Many of us travel through each day without thinking about this loving core within us, and sometimes we feel alone, exhausted, and old. To avoid this unpleasant state, we just need to recognize that sacred energy is always available to us from both within and without. Once we acknowledge this, we then can move spiritually, mentally, emotionally, and physically into its natural, ever-present flow. We can hold the intention of actively working with it and being surrounded by its rejuvenating peace and beauty.

Today's world, which bombards us with information, presents us with many choices of how to lead our lives. So why not choose to act on proven, available techniques that will bring us joy, peace, and physical energy, giving us the enthusiasm of a young child learning a new game?

If you and I practice the carefully outlined spiritual, mental, emotional, and physical steps suggested in *Ancient Secrets of Facial Rejuvenation*, we will tap into the flow of positive energy, both internal and external, in a big way. We will experience the peace, health, and love that we were meant to enjoy as human beings.

Doing the Acupressure Facelift exercises in this book will provide you with valuable practice in tuning in to the personal and the universal energy source. You will find yourself expressing the inner flow of your energy outwardly, sending it to others through a youthful face that projects and reflects only your deep feelings of contentment and well-being. This practice can also open the way to a wonderful new level of physical health.

You will discover that others will want to learn the secrets behind your youthful well-being. They will feel so good just being around you that they will insist on hearing how you became the new, rejuvenated you. Of course, at that point, you will smile lovingly . . . and tell them your secret.

The information that is so clearly presented in this book will provide you with everything you need to activate the inner and outer miracle of beauty and well-being. It is exciting and empowering to know that this life-enhancing information is now available to us all. It is even more rewarding to realize that Victoria Mogilner's methods are a noninvasive way to achieve incredible good for ourselves at our own pace. What a gift!

— Angela M. Mattey, author of
Table Tipping: The Key to Spiritual and Psychic Development

Preface

When I was a child, I wasn't very sure of myself. I felt klutzy. I was afraid of not doing things right; therefore, I didn't trust myself. As I moved into adulthood, I continued to lack poise and self-confidence.

I was first exposed to Chinese medicine in my twenties as a client. During that time, I was living in England and met my teacher and practitioner, Dr. Worsley. His treatments helped me emotionally, physically, and spiritually; they brought me a sense of balance and helped me to gain my inner confidence. I was a client for four years and then chose to study acupuncture because it works on an emotional and spiritual level and focuses on the causes of illness, rather than the symptoms. During the course of my studies, I learned about the concepts of longevity and renewal. I began to see that as we age, we need to take care of ourselves from the inside out through diet, exercise, and attitude. I realized that beauty, as they say, is only skin deep.

I was so impressed with Eastern philosophy that I began applying its principles to my life. I was doing tai chi, watching my diet — eating warm, nurturing foods — and taking charge of my emotional needs. I started living in harmony with the seasons: taking time for personal renewal in the winter, planning direction for my life in the spring, being more active in the summer, and gathering my inner harvest of plans and decisions in the late summer and autumn. The poise and self-confidence that I had been missing began to seep into my pores.

Later, in my work as an acupuncturist, I was exposed to facial rejuvenation, a practice based on Chinese medicine, and I received some treatments to experience it firsthand. The basic idea behind it is that by using specific acupressure techniques, one can look and feel younger. I was amazed at how renewed and balanced I felt. My skin felt tight and replenished. I decided to study facial rejuvenation and incorporate it into my practice and life. As I was further exposed to this new concept and as I became professionally engaged in facial acupressure, I saw that I had been wearing a mask of facial expressions and mannerisms that reflected my self-doubt and insecurity, the old, negative patterns I had carried with me from childhood. I could also see that this mask was dropping away; I no longer wore a frown or had trouble looking people in the eyes. I continued to gain self-assurance and feel more comfortable in my body.

What I love most about facial rejuvenation is that it balances the whole person. By touching the right points, we can clear away old emotions and influence our physical and mental health. As I received these treatments, I saw a radiance emerge from inside me. My skin glowed, and my eyes became clear. Worry and fear left my body. I felt replenished. The negative patterns left over from my childhood were melting away. As I delved further into facial rejuvenation, I learned that change is an ongoing process and that there are no short-cuts to growth. At first, though, I needed to be reminded of these things constantly, so every time I looked at my face in a mirror or in any shiny surface, I said a special affirmation: *I love myself the way I am, with all my perfections and imperfections.*

As I embraced all of me, I became a much more integrated person. And by having compassion for myself, I gradually learned that I could also have compassion for others. I saw quite clearly that I could not love another until I learned to love and appreciate myself. Certainly, I could not give anything of real value to anyone else until I gave something to me. I found that emotional scarring and baggage from the early years could be transformed through self-love and nourishment and that believing in myself was the first step toward loving myself.

As I felt myself becoming transformed through the wondrous techniques of Chinese facial rejuvenation, my passion for these healing techniques grew. I wanted to give this gift to others.

I believe that this book will give you the opportunity to come home to yourself, to understand who you really are. By doing the exercises included here daily, you will be giving yourself the time to see yourself and your life in a new way. I trust that you will learn, as I have, that being present, rather than thinking of the past or the future, will allow you to deepen your connection with your essence.

My wish for you is that you will not simply employ the Acupressure Facelift to create a more youthful appearance, but that you will use it to learn to truly love every inch, every cell, of your being. I believe that you will discover a deeper, more satisfying connection with your own soul and gain the fullness of life you have always yearned for.

Introduction

We are living in a time, particularly in the United States, of unparalleled focus on physical beauty. We are judged for the way we look and encouraged to change any aspect of our being that may not measure up to the unattainable ideals we see on the pages of magazines. Further, this is a time of almost unlimited opportunity to "improve" our appearance through innumerable surgical, chemical, and laser procedures. It is no secret that more and more of us are racing to plastic surgeons and specialized clinics, where all our so-called deficiencies can be corrected.

All but completely obscured by these latest techniques is an age-old approach to facial rejuvenation that is natural and nurturing, one that achieves the same results as the modern techniques. Handed down from Chinese medicine, it is known as Acupressure Facial Rejuvenation. I call it the Acupressure Facelift. It is a nonsurgical and painless method of erasing years from the face, but it is much more than just a cosmetic procedure. The Facelift is a rejuvenation and revitalization process designed to help the whole body look and feel younger. When you enter the world of Chinese medicine via the Acupressure Facelift, you will open a doorway to health care on the mental, physical, and spiritual levels.

Acupressure is a Chinese practice of lightly pressing specific points on the body with the tips of the fingers. Acupressure can be performed by a practitioner, or you can do it to yourself. When you press on the acupressure points, energy flows to them, stimulating blood flow and improving circulation. The acupressure techniques in this book teach you to touch yourself with love, taking time for yourself each morning and setting the tone of the day.

As you touch your face and throat, you influence your life mentally, physically, and emotionally by giving your body a very important message of self-love and pampering. The brain receives the message to relax and slow down and relays it throughout your body. Then your emotions balance and you can let go of anger, fear, and depression. Instead you feel invigorated and nurtured.

Ancient Secrets of Facial Rejuvenation is a practical guide to working on your face — and your whole self — from the inside out. It will teach you the secret of longevity, to which there are no shortcuts. It will also give you tips on how to eat, exercise, use nature's remedies such as essential oils, live in harmony with the seasons, and replenish yourself. By following a daily rhythm and observing nature you will have tools to stay balanced.

You may easily turn to any section of this book and learn how to receive many benefits, including smoother facial skin, improved circulation, and enhanced self-appreciation. The chapters are organized as follows:

- Chapter 1 looks at some of the fundamentals of Chinese medicine, which are the cornerstones of the Acupressure Facelift.

- Chapter 2 offers basic information about the skin, including the various skin types and common causes of skin damage.

- Chapter 3 covers the preliminaries of the Facelift, such as the Prefacial Warm-up, a description of the various components of the Facelift, and the guidelines for performing the Facelift.

- Chapter 4 presents the Facelift itself, comprising thirteen acupressure points.

- Chapter 5 explores how acupressure can be used to treat other common maladies that show up in the face — from stomach cramps to irregular heartbeats.

- Chapter 6 offers an overview of the fundamentals of healthy nutrition from the Chinese perspective. Eating a balanced diet according to these guidelines is another piece of the skin-care puzzle.

- Chapter 7 considers the importance of living in tune with the seasons and offers suggestions to do so.

- Chapter 8 looks at another skin- and health-care gift from Mother Nature, essential oils, which can be used to treat the skin, the rest of the body, the mind, and the spirit.

- Chapter 9 concludes the book with a look at additional elements of a healthy, balanced lifestyle, such as the Chinese practices of *qigong* and tai chi , the Hawaiian spirit of Aloha, the importance of proper rest, techniques of self-massage, and the power of positive thinking.

The Acupressure Facelift, as well as the other rejuvenation techniques covered in this book, facilitates transformation, for it opens doorways to new ideas, new methods of self-expression, and a deeper, more nurturing relationship with yourself. You will come to understand that beauty is only skin deep and will gain tools to go deeper into yourself to bring your life into balance and relieve stress.

As you adopt these practices, you will replenish at the cellular level, enabling you to shift away from old attitudes and beliefs that constrict your life. In their place you will learn to create peace of mind. Most important, perhaps, is that while engaging these techniques, you will be learning to love and appreciate your essence. You will be sending a sense of well-being to every pore, and your body will say, "Thank you for taking care of me." You will have the tools to guide your life toward wholeness.

You may use this practical guide as a how-to book for facial renewal as well as spiritual renewal. It will help you to stay healthy, change your attitude, regenerate yourself, and live a blissful life in harmony with nature.

ANCIENT
SECRETS OF
FACIAL
REJUVENATION

CHAPTER ONE

Facial Rejuvenation and the Oldest Medical System

M ost of us have been taught the maxim "love thy neighbor as thyself." But the great practitioners of Chinese medicine teach that you cannot love another until you first love yourself, and you cannot give to others what you cannot give to yourself. More fundamentally, you cannot know who and what you are until you take the time to tune in to your inner self. Listening to yourself and giving to yourself are the pathways to self-love, and there are no shortcuts to it.

While growing up, most of us were never taught how to love ourselves in a way that truly nurtures our physical body, our emotional self, or — especially — our spiritual essence. And we spend so many of our adult years unlearning the rules and concepts we once thought valid. But when we finally do learn to take care of ourselves, we are empowered to attain greater health and wholeness, and we are provided with the capacity to truly care for others. In order to feel and exude our true self, we must let go of an often painful past; we must shift old attitudes that constrict, and instead learn to create peace of mind.

Being beautiful is an "inside job," which takes time to cultivate, just like a garden. As you plant thoughts of self-love, you take time to connect with your soul and spirit. Love, healing, joy, peace, tranquility, and gratefulness are the nutrients for your spiritual growth. This inner gardening requires going within daily to replenish and connect with your spiritual essence. When you set aside time each day for yourself, your work within will be reflected without. The techniques you will find in this book will give you the tools you need do that inner work to achieve inner balance, beauty, and harmony.

This chapter lays the groundwork for the rest of the book. It presents the fundamentals of Chinese medicine, including an explanation of its major principles, such as chi and the meridians. With this background information, you will be equipped to begin reaping the benefits of the Acupressure Facelift.

The Traditions and Philosophy of Chinese Medicine

Chinese medicine, more than three thousand years old, is the most ancient medical system in the world. Its philosophy is that you pay the doctor when you are well, and the doctor pays you when you become ill. This maxim illustrates the preventive nature of Chinese medicine. As you learn to take care of yourself and practice preventive medicine by eating a healthy diet, getting proper exercise, keeping a positive attitude, living in tune with the seasons, and practicing the acupressure and other techniques in this book, you can prevent many illnesses and learn to be healthy and content.

Chinese medicine is concerned with restoring balance throughout the body and promoting the flow of energy, which is called *chi* (pronounced "chee"). Chi is the life force that represents your strong spirit. When I use the term *chi* I am speaking of your vital essence, which can be reflected in your eyes, for in Chinese philosophy, we say the eyes are the gateway to the soul. When your eyes are bright, your chi is vital and alive.

Chi is circulated along a subtle energy system, a transportation network consisting of channels, usually called meridians. There are fourteen meridians in the body, each relating to one of the vital organs. So that you can better visualize the concept of chi and the meridians, think of the meridians as a riverbed and the chi as the water that flows through it and nourishes the land. If a dam were placed at any point along the river, the nourishing effect of the water would be blocked. The same is true of the meridians and chi. When the chi becomes blocked along a meridian in one area, the rest of the body suffers. Illness and disease can result if the flow is not restored.

In traditional Chinese medicine, a well-known maxim states "If there is pain, there is no free flow. If there is free flow, there is no pain." Healthy individuals experience a free flow of their chi and blood. Chinese medicine removes obstacles so that chi and blood flow smoothly, restoring balance and correct function. Practitioners of Chinese medicine recognize that there is no "one size fits all" therapy for an interruption of chi, just as they know that identical symptoms can result from entirely different root causes. They use four primary treatment methods to restore balance, approaches designed to treat the whole person: diet, herbal medicinal formulas, acupuncture/acupressure, and massage, all of which will be covered in this book.

Chi and blood flow through the body at certain times during the day, so in order to live a long life, it is important to follow certain guidelines that reflect the body's cycles and optimal functioning. Establishing a regular rhythm and living with the cycles of nature will keep you healthy, and simple scheduling patterns will keep you young. Keys to longevity include: early to bed, early to rise; eating lightly and at regular hours; being active by day and resting after sundown; and breathing life into each and every cell. Leisurely walks in spring, sunbaths in summer, stretching the body in all seasons, watching the mind each moment, avoiding anger, and living easy — all are critical to replenishing the self from the inside to the outside.

Nei Ching, the ancient book on Chinese philosophy and medicine, gives us the fundamentals for living a full life. Inherent in its teachings is that longevity and rejuvenation are partly states of mind that depend heavily on one's connection to the divine life force. When connected to spirituality, one is less likely to be a victim of life's circumstances.

Another important concept in Chinese medicine is that of *yin* and *yang*. Yin and yang represent the duality of the universe. They are the cosmic forces of creative energy. Yin refers to your softer, female side, which relates to taking time for you, flowing with life, and not being hard on or judgmental of yourself. It means going within to replenish and recharge. Yang refers to the body's active, masculine energy, characterized as hard, bright, and overpowering. Yang can manifest as being aggressive, loud, and out of control — running around all the time and being obnoxious and unruly. The balance between yin and yang is what we strive for in our lives. Yin and yang are interdependent as well as conflicting. In traditional Chinese medicine their relationship is used to explain the physiology and pathology of the human body, and it refers to your lifestyle as well as your constitution.

Yin also relates to your internal organs, called *Zang Fu* — your liver, spleen, kidneys, heart, and lungs. The health of these organs is reflected in the color in your face, and we'll learn more about this in chapter 5. Any imbalances in your organs can be corrected with proper diet, exercise, and lifestyle, as well as work on your facial points.

Remember, the outside reflects the inside; everything you do shows on your face. When you learn to take care of yourself on the inside, it will show — you will have glowing skin, a sparkle in your eyes, and a calm presence.

The Meridians and the Acupressure Facelift

As mentioned above, there are a total of fourteen meridians, twelve primary meridians and two other major meridians called the Conception Vessel and Governor Vessel. Each of the meridians corresponds to an internal organ, as well as an emotion, with the exception of the Conception Vessel and the Governor Vessel. These are not connected to any single organ or emotion but instead are the "mommy and daddy" that give birth to the other twelve meridians. The Conception Vessel, the most yin meridian, starts at the perineum (the lowest point of the pubic bone) and runs up the center of the body, ending under the mouth on the chin. The Governor Vessel, the most yang meridian, starts at the coccyx, or base of the spine, and runs up the midline of the back and over the top of the head to a spot just above the upper lip. The Conception Vessel and Governor Vessel connect under the tongue.

Like the two major meridians, most of the others begin or end on the face. Thus, when you touch the points on your face included in the Acupressure Facelift, you will be positively affecting many other parts of your body as well.

The Meridian Clock

In Chinese medicine, each of the twelve major organs has a two-hour period of high energy and a two-hour period of low energy. The meridian clock shown on the next page illustrates this concept. Working with an organ, or the meridian related to it, during its high-energy period always reaps the greatest benefits, while during the low-energy period, the organ is resting. For example, if you want to work on digestion, it is best to do it during the stomach's most active time, 8:00 a.m.

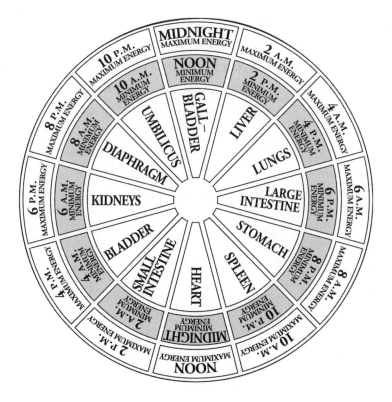

The negative emotion associated with the stomach is worry or overthinking, while its positive emotion is self-nurturing. So, if you want to release worry or stress and foster self-nurturing, the most effective approach would be to work on the stomach at 8:00 a.m. You could visualize letting go of stress and bringing nourishment into your life. Affirmations, positive thoughts stated as affirmative sentences, are very effective with this type of work; for this example, a useful affirmation could be, "I release all my worries to my higher self, and I bring nourishment to every cell of my being." Saying this affirmation would be a good way to start your day.

You can work on all your organs in this way via the meridians that begin and end on your face. You will learn how to do this in chapter 4, which presents the Acupressure Facelift in detail.

WHEN YOU APPLY THE WISDOM of Chinese medicine to skin care, your face will respond by appearing more healthy and radiant. The next chapter presents some fundamentals about the skin.

CHAPTER TWO

Toward a More Youthful Face

Everything you think and everything you feel is reflected on your face. And every line you see there is related to an emotional or physical condition in your body.

What others see on your face depends on many factors in your life. If you live in isolation, the shadows of loneliness, sadness, and depression are revealed on your face. But as you create a life of joy, harmony, and fulfillment, the positive effects of these gifts will emerge there instead.

Since every point on your face has a spiritual and physical meaning, when you touch your face, you connect directly with your spiritual essence. You can help release fear, depression, and anger by looking into the mirror and gently touching your face. You can heal old traumas and wounds and help create a new life of joy and love.

Through regular use of the Acupressure Facelift, you can become more closely and deeply connected to the divine spirit at your core. As you learn to recognize the truth that comes from your inner divinity, you can make choices that will help you achieve the best for your physical, mental, and spiritual well-being.

To prepare you for this transformational practice, this chapter presents some basic information about the skin, including its function, the various skin types, some common causes of skin damage, and how the Acupressure Facelift works to revitalize the skin.

Skin Fundamentals

The skin is the largest organ of the body. Governed by the lungs, it influences all other body systems, helping the other organs to recharge and de-stress, and the immune system to strengthen. When you take care of your facial skin, you also help your internal organs, for the health of your organs shows on your face.

The skin is comprised of seven layers. The five outermost layers are called the epidermis; they are what you feel when you touch your skin, put on makeup, or shave. Through a process called keratinization (so named because it is activated by the fibrous protein keratin), cells are continually being formed at the innermost layer of the epidermis and moved outward, layer by layer, until they are finally sloughed off. For any given epidermal cell, this process takes about thirty days.

However, damage to skin fibers interferes with the process of cell renewal and is the primary cause of wrinkles and aging.

Beneath the epidermis is the dermis, which actually has two layers containing the connective tissue, blood, and lymph to supply nourishment for the skin. This is where the sweat and oil glands are located. The deepest layer of the dermis gives the skin its elasticity and strength. Collagen, a protein, makes up 90 percent of the dermis.

The skin performs six vital functions:

Protection: The skin acts as a barrier to protect the body's tissues from dehydration and to prevent invasion from harmful organisms. The skin also produces melanin, an enzyme that blocks the sun's ultraviolet rays.

Sensation: The skin contains innumerable nerve endings that make it sensitive to heat and cold, as well as to pressure, vibration, and injury.

Temperature control: The skin regulates body temperature. In cold weather, blood vessels contract to conserve heat, and the hairs on the skin trap a layer of heat to provide insulation. In hot weather, the blood vessels dilate to allow heat to escape.

Storage and synthesis: The skin stores water and lipids (various fatty compounds), and it synthesizes vitamins B and D when activated by the ultraviolet rays of the sun.

Absorption: Important gases such as oxygen, nitrogen, and carbon dioxide are absorbed by the skin in small amounts.

Also, the skin can absorb healing substances, such as aloe vera and essential oils, that are found in lotions and ointments.

Waste removal: Sweat glands in the skin function both to help control body temperature and to remove toxic substances, such as urea, from the body.

Proper diet, healthy exercise, and adequate hydration all play a major role in natural skin care. By drinking eight glasses of room-temperature water every day; eating warm, nurturing foods; and touching your face with love, you can help replenish your cells and therefore keep your skin healthy, alive, and vital. If you appreciate your appearance, your cells will respond and send a message to the brain, which will help with rejuvenation and skin repair. Remember, the more you maintain your skin, the healthier it will stay.

Skin Types and How to Treat Them

There are five types of skin: normal, dry, oily, sensitive, and combination. Normal skin is neither too dry, too oily, nor too rough and may be affected by climate, hormonal problems, or stress.

Dry skin is caused by too much wind, harsh soaps, poor diet, and insufficient fluid intake. The skin becomes dry due to inactivity of the sebaceous glands that lubricate the skin. Since it has less oil, dry skin is more prone to wrinkles and lines. If you have dry skin, it helps to use a rich moisturizing cream; eating foods high in Omega-3 fatty acids, such as salmon, trout, and flax seed will also help. Avoid too much sun and wind. For dry to normal skin, use a light scrub (a honey or almond scrub works well) two or three times a week to get rid of dead skin and help the skin to breathe.

Oily skin usually indicates an excess of internal heat in your system; typically, the pores get clogged more easily, resulting in blackheads, whiteheads, and enlarged pores. If you have oily skin, use water-based products. Make sure your hands are clean before you touch your face so you don't increase the oiliness. Removing dead cells with a gentle exfoliant is helpful in treating oily and acne-prone skin.

If you have sensitive skin, you should avoid harsh soaps and instead use a gentle cleansing milk. Use moisturizers containing calming ingredients, such as aloe vera or chamomile. Avoid spicy foods and alcohol, for these may aggravate your condition. Always wash your hands before touching your face, and be sure to touch your face gently.

In combination skin, the forehead, nose, and chin (known as the T-zone) are oily and the rest of the face is dry or normal. To balance combination skin, minimize fat and oil in your diet. Also, it is best to use an oil-free moisturizer, for this will hydrate the skin without adding excess oils that could exacerbate the oiliness in the T-zone. If you have combination skin, you may also want to treat the T-zone separately, with products designed for oily skin.

Mature, aging, or sun-damaged skin needs antioxidants — such as vitamins C and E and grape seed extract — either applied topically or taken orally. The goal here is to hydrate the skin and help it to firm. Getting facials will also help aging or sun-damaged skin, as will a positive attitude.

In chapter 6, we'll learn about healthy nutrition for the different skin types.

Causes of Skin Damage

Skin is influenced by heredity, sun exposure, the environment, health habits, hormones, and lifestyle. You cannot change your heredity, certainly, but you can do a great deal about all these other factors. Damage to the skin is not inevitable, not simply a matter of time. Your biological clock is, of course, a factor, and skin shows the signs of aging most visibly. Lines begin to show, and gravity eventually causes the skin to sag. Skin-care experts agree that this happens because, over time, the skin loses its ability to produce necessary oils. Nevertheless, there is much you can do to slow or even reverse many of the causes of skin damage. To maintain the best possible youthful appearance, you should avoid the following dangers to your skin.

Sun Exposure

After heredity, the sun and its ultraviolet rays have the greatest impact on skin. There are two different types of ultraviolet radiation contained in the sun's rays; these are known as UVA and UVB. The first

type, UVA, is also called the "aging ray." It weakens the skin's collagen and elastic fibers, causing wrinkling and sagging. UVB rays,
meanwhile, are the "burning rays" and affect the cells of the epidermis — the top layer of the skin that produces melanin. Melanin protects the skin from the sun's UV rays, but it can be altered or
destroyed when skin is exposed to the sun for a long period. So it is
important to not spend a lot of time in the sun; if you do, your skin will
become weathered and dried as you get older. Even if you think you
are not out in the sun very much, you need to wear a sunscreen with
a sun protective factor (SPF) of 15 or more on all exposed areas.

Pollution

Pollution from car exhaust and secondhand smoke can affect the
health of the skin as well as the underlying cells and tissues. The best
way to protect skin from pollution is to wash it every night with warm
water and to gently exfoliate any dead skin cells that have settled on
the surface. Using a moisturizer will also help protect the skin.

When cleansing the face, do not use soap, since doing so strips
the top layer, known as the acid mantle. The best guide in picking
a cleansing product is to note how it feels on your face. A good
cleanser should remove impurities and loosen skin cells. A moisturizer should be absorbed easily and not leave a greasy film. Before
buying a product, read its list of ingredients and know what function
each of the ingredients performs.

Tobacco, Alcohol, and Other Drugs

Poor lifestyle habits can also harm the skin. Smoking tobacco, for example, has been linked to premature aging and wrinkling. The nicotine in tobacco causes contraction and weakening of the blood vessels and capillaries that supply blood to the body's tissues, causing decreased circulation. Smokers' skin can appear yellow or gray.

Drinking alcohol is another habit that is harmful to the skin. It can dilate the blood vessels and capillaries, weakening their walls. This in turn can cause the skin to appear flushed. Alcohol can also dehydrate skin by drawing water out of its cells, which causes the skin to appear dry. In the same way, many other drugs can interfere with the body's intake of oxygen and can cause dryness.

Dehydration

Water comprises about 65 percent of the body's weight. Even mild dehydration slows the metabolism and can cause fatigue. Further, dehydration can cause the skin to feel sluggish and leathery. Therefore, drink at least eight glasses of room-temperature water daily. This will aid in the elimination of toxins and waste and promote proper digestion.

Poor Nutrition

Poor eating habits, such as eating on the run and eating processed and fast foods, can clog pores. In contrast, getting the proper nutrition will feed cells, help with collagen production, and help cells to repair damage. The skin is nourished by the blood and lymph flowing through the arteries and capillaries. The foods you eat and the water you drink are your body's basic building blocks. In fact, your body is like a machine, and all of its parts depend on the foods you eat to function properly.

In the tradition of Chinese medicine, we talk about a balance of the five flavors: a little salt to feed the kidneys, a little sour to feed the liver and gallbladder, a little pungent to feed the lungs and large intestine (also known as the colon), a little sweet to feed the stomach and spleen, and a little bitter to feed the heart and small intestine. The law of Chinese medicine is moderation. Eating too much of anything can injure the body. For example, too much heat in your system from eating spicy foods can create a hormonal imbalance. This can irritate the skin, causing redness and dryness. Choosing warm and nurturing foods, eating slowly, and avoiding serious emotional discussions while eating will all aid the digestive process. You will learn more about supporting the skin with proper nutrition in chapter 6.

Adolescence, Menopause, and Other Hormonal Changes

Hormonal imbalances and changes can cause acne and clog the pores. In turn, the sebaceous glands will produce more sebum, and pores will dilate farther. Therefore, cleansing the skin properly is critical.

Because of the abrupt hormonal changes of adolescence, teenagers, in particular, need good skin-care education. Teenagers should eliminate fried foods and be taught how to properly cleanse their skin so as to not clog their pores with too much makeup.

During menopause, many women experience mood swings and have flushed, dry, itchy, and tired-looking skin. Menopausal hot flashes are caused by a fluctuation of blood flow due to hormonal changes. Herbs such as black cohosh, which is available at herbal stores and can be made into a tea or taken in capsules, may help balance the endocrine system, the system that produces these hormones. Additionally, inhaling the essential oil ylang ylang will help balance hormones, since it stimulates the pituitary gland, which regulates the hormonal cycle. Practicing tai chi can also help balance the pathways (see chapter 9 for more on tai chi), which will aid in decreasing moodiness and increasing the oxygen exchange that will help replenish skin.

Stress and Painful Emotions

When you are unhappy or stressed out, it will show on your face. Stress can affect the hormonal cycle, causing constriction of the blood vessels and affecting the liver, which can result in the appearance of crow's feet around the eyes. Succumbing to anger can dilate blood vessels and break capillaries. Fear can affect the adrenals and cause skin to look weathered and worn. Worry and anxiety can age skin by making it look sallow and pasty.

On the other hand, staying connected to your inner essence will keep you youthful, help give you a positive attitude, and keep you centered during stressful periods in your life. Avoiding spicy foods, eating more soy, balancing your hormones with exercise, breathing deeply, meditating, exercising, and drinking enough water will all help steady hormonal and emotional changes. Your skin will have a healthy glow when you are emotionally balanced and content.

The Acupressure Facelift and Its Benefits

Avoiding the dangers to your skin discussed above and using natural herbal products and essential oils will tighten and replenish your skin. We are now ready to add to these practices the Acupressure Facelift. The Facelift is not just a process for looking better. It is a system for total rejuvenation of the body, mind, and spirit.

Many of the meridians you learned about in chapter 1 begin or end with points on the face. When the meridians are blocked, the aging process is accelerated, causing the skin on the face to look dull. Moreover, when the meridians become clogged through improper diet, negative emotions (which shut down the cells), and lack of water, skin can age prematurely and systems can shut down. But when these pathways are opened, they are like flowing rivers, and you become rejuvenated, refreshed, recharged, and replenished. Your body feels youthful; you are bright and alert; your face glows.

Working on the face opens the meridian pathways throughout your body. Your skin will glow and become more elastic as a result, and you will be accomplishing many things in the whole body, such as:

- aiding digestion and the assimilation of nutrients;

- improving hearing;

- helping the back to stay healthy and strong;

- improving the circulation in the face and body by replenishing blood and energy;

- stimulating the lymphatic system, which is like an irrigation system that drains waste, bacteria, and toxins from tissues;

- assisting the immune system to stay healthy.

Most important, perhaps, is that while using these techniques you will be learning to love and appreciate your essence. The effects of these treatments will be increased if you work on yourself regularly with patience, love, and attention focused on your desired outcome.

Now you are ready to learn about the Facelift. In the next chapter, you will do just that.

CHAPTER THREE

Setting the Stage
for the Acupressure Facelift

In this chapter you will find all the information you need to pave the way for your Acupressure Facelift routine. First we will consider some preliminaries, such as setting aside a sacred time and place for your practice, and the Prefacial Warm-up. Then we will learn about the components of the practice and the guidelines for treatment.

Sacred Time and Space

Chinese medicine teaches that a healing treatment should be a sacred time of spiritual renewal. This time is sacred, because you are sacred. As you set aside a period each day for spiritual renewal, realize that your surroundings are an important part of the picture. Choose a space where you can sit comfortably, focus on your breathing, and reduce the distractions of daily life. Create a setting conducive to your spiritual work, a sacred space filled with flickering candlelight and the sounds of soft, meditative music. And set aside a specific time each day for your journey of self-discovery. You will begin to feel the benefits almost immediately.

Start each day by setting a spiritual, physical, and emotional intention for yourself and visualizing what you want to receive and experience that day.

Taking short breaks throughout the day will help to replenish you. These minibreaks might involve nothing more than closing your eyes and breathing deeply. As you connect with your essence throughout the day, you will be recharged.

At the end of the day, ask yourself what you need to do to nurture yourself, perhaps by giving yourself a massage or listening to soothing music. Additionally, review your day. Write a gratitude list, naming all the day's happenings or influences that you are grateful for. And take time to look within to see where you could have been more aware, loving, or conscious that day.

The Prefacial Warm-Up

Just as you should warm up your muscles before exercising, you should prepare yourself for your Acupressure Facelift by becoming completely relaxed. Performed regularly each day, the following four-minute warm-up will help you to receive maximum benefits for your efforts. It will relax you and will set the tone for nurturing yourself.

During the warm-up and the Facelift itself, sit in a place where you feel safe, tranquil, and nurtured. Begin to breathe steadily, and picture every part of your body — every pore, every cell — receiving nourishment. Sit quietly and reflect on your life. Still your mind, and come to see the beauty inside you. Relax and enjoy.

Remain focused on your breath. As you breathe out, let go of stress. As you breathe in, repeat to yourself your intention for the day; you can use the affirmation, "I let go of old thoughts. I work on myself to replenish myself at the cellular level," or you can make up an affirmation of your own.

The following steps will relax and prepare different parts of your body for the Facelift. It's best to perform the steps in order and to do them for one minute each before embarking on your Facelift treatment.

1. For Circulation to the Head and Face

Press your thumbs gently into both sides of your collarbone and hold for one minute. Take a deep breath in through the nose, then exhale slowly through the mouth. Relax and move your hands gently upward, working on either side of the throat area. You are stimulating the thymus, bringing circulation to the front of the face and setting the tone for a relaxing, healing experience.

Helping Hands

For step 2A of the Prefacial Warm-up, as well as several of the techniques in chapter 5, you will need what I refer to as "Helping Hands." These are devices that you can place on a flat surface, such as a floor or the back of chair, and then lie or lean back on to stimulate the pressure points in your back. You have a couple of options of what to use as your Helping Hands. My favorite is to take a tennis ball or a dog ball (a small rubber ball available at pet stores) and to cut it in half; the two halves will function as two Helping Hands. Alternatively, you can tie a hand towel in a knot and use the knot as your Helping Hand. You'll be amazed at how these help to release tension in places your own hands can't reach.

2. For Tension in the Shoulders and Upper Back

Exercise A: Sit on the floor and place two Helping Hands on the floor behind you. Lie down, positioning the Helping Hands under each of your shoulder blades. Release control and feel your shoulders relax while you focus your thoughts on letting go of both physical tension and emotions that are no longer relevant in your life. Lie there for one minute, breathing deeply. Relax before moving on to the next step.

Exercise B: Lie flat on your back, place your fingers under your head, and gently press your thumbs into the sides of the base of your skull. Hold for one minute, breathing deeply. Be sure to visualize your arms at ease. Relax and continue breathing. As you press into this particular point, you are stimulating your eyes. Focus on inner strength, inner self-control, and a new inner vision.

3. For Tension in the Jaw

Let your jaw hang open. Rest your index and middle fingers on the front sides of your forehead, and press your thumbs deeply into the indentation at the jaw hinges for one minute. As you begin to work with this point, reflect on what you intend to let go of in your life and what you need for inner healing and circulation. You are releasing tension in the jaw and throat center in order to be open to the inspiration that will come as you work on yourself.

NOW IT'S TIME to learn more about the Facelift.

> Reading the steps of the Acupressure Facelift thoroughly before treating any of the points will allow you to understand the physical process as well as the mental and spiritual benefits that each point can provide.

Components of the Acupressure Facelift

The Facelift consists of thirteen acupressure points. All of the points are presented in the next chapter in a consistent format so you can follow along easily; the description of each point includes the following elements:

Meridian: Each point lies along a specific meridian and effects the related organ.

Meaning of name: Each point has a name, translated into English from Chinese. The names may sound strange at first, so I include an explanation of each name's meaning and origin. Knowing the name of a given point and keeping it in mind as you treat it will contribute to the treatment's effectiveness.

Position: This includes the physical position of the point on the face and, in parentheses, the numbered location of the point on the related meridian.

Physical benefits: Treating each point promotes specific physical benefits in the body by releasing tension and improving circulation.

Spiritual benefits: Likewise, each point has the power to enhance aspects of your spiritual well-being.

Best time of day: Treating a point during the high-energy period of the related organ (see the Meridian Clock on page 9) will help you reap the greatest benefits. However, the peak times for some points are in the middle of the night, while others may fall during the busiest time of your workday, so it may not be possible to treat every point during its high-energy period. Whenever you can, do treat points during their high-energy periods, and when you can't, don't worry too much about it — treating the points at any time of the day produces glowing results.

How-to: This section includes detailed instructions on how to position your fingers on the point.

Essential oil: For each point, certain essential oils can help open the energy pathways so you receive the greatest benefit.

Suggested affirmation: With each technique, I have included an affirmation, or positive thought, that you may use as a point of focus. Or you may make up your own affirmations.

Special application: Touching the points on your face can help initiate new phases in your life, invoke specific conditions you'd like to manifest, and release those things that are no longer working for you. For some of the points I include ideas for these kinds of special treatments.

Guidelines for Performing the Acupressure Facelift

To achieve the best results, follow these guidelines when performing the Facelift:

- Take time for the warm-up and the Facelift each morning first thing upon rising. Set aside five minutes for the warm-up and ten minutes or more for the Facelift. To start with, choose one or two points to treat each day. As you become more experienced with the Facelift, you may wish to spend more time and treat more points so you can go deeper within yourself and allow for a greater transformation.

- Treat the points in the areas of your face that most concern you. To achieve maximum benefits for problem areas, you may treat them three consecutive times during a single session.

- As you perform the Facelift, breathe deeply, focusing your attention on the point you're treating. Visualize sending love to the point, as well as letting go of stress, anxiety, or any emotion you wish to release.

- As you press on a specific point, depending on which feels more comfortable to you, you may use only your index finger or the pads of all your fingers. The key is your focus and intention. You will be opening the meridian pathway and linking it to its corresponding organ for healing and balance.

- Do not be overly concerned about finding the exact point. Your body is like a network — each point affects other points along the pathway. The effects are cumulative, and as you do more self-treatment and become sensitive to energy flow, your finger will instinctively go to the correct points. As long as you are in the general area, you will affect each point.

- Touch and then hold each point with steady, gentle pressure on both sides of your face. Release after one minute.

- You may alternate gradual pressure and release. As you do this several times, you will be releasing old negative thought patterns.

- You may rotate your fingertips in small circular movements to help replenish each point. Rotating clockwise brings energy to a point and releases blocked energy.

- Take care not to stretch or pull your skin, for the skin on the face is delicate.

NOW YOU ARE READY TO LEARN the thirteen points of the Facelift. The next chapter presents them in detail.

CHAPTER FOUR

The Acupressure Facelift: A Step-by-Step Practice

This chapter explores the Accupressure Facelift, step by step. The chart on the following pages lists the names of the points and shows where each is located. The name of the meridian stimulated by the point appears in parentheses. You may want to use this as a quick-reference guide as you become familiar with the techniques of the Facelift.

Following the chart, we'll look at each point in detail. You may notice that many of the points — six out of thirteen — relate to the stomach meridian. This is because the stomach and the face are closely connected; the stomach is the meridian with the most points on the face. Keep this in mind when you make dietary decisions, for the results of those decisions can show up on your face.

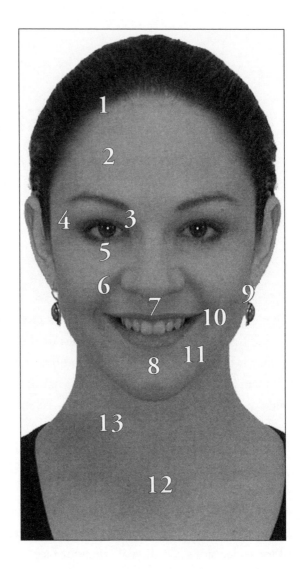

1. Skulls Safeguard (Stomach)

2. Yang Brightness (Gallbladder)

3. Eyes Bright (Bladder)

4. Pupil Bone (Gallbladder)

5. Receiving Cures (Stomach)

6. Welcome Fragrance (Colon)

7. Middle Man (Governor Vessel)

8. Receiving Fluids (Conception Vessel)

9. Lower Hinge (Stomach)

10. Stomach Granary (Stomach)

11. Mandible Wheel (Stomach)

12. Angel Spring (Conception Vessel)

13. Greeting Welcome (Stomach)

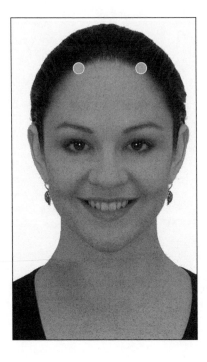

1. Skulls Safeguard

Meridian: Stomach

Meaning of name: The name of this point refers to feeling safe and being nurtured, since the stomach relates to internal security and self-nourishment.

Position: Hairline, directly above the eyes (position 8 along the stomach meridian)

Physical benefits: Helps with frontal headaches and overthinking.

Spiritual benefits: Helps to release past trauma, easing turmoil to promote inner peace. Opens up new self-perceptions and possibilities for your role in the world.

Best time of day: 7:00–9:00 a.m. (8:00 a.m. is the peak time).

How-to: Place your thumbs or fingers along the corners of the forehead, one half inch from the hairline or straight up from the highest point of your eyebrow. Press upward and hold for a count of sixty seconds, breathing gently.

As you apply pressure you are helping your forehead to relax. If you are tied up in knots you may first envision what you are holding on to and then envision releasing it. As you work with this point, think about releasing the past generally and discontinuing your old patterns of negative thinking. Allow yourself to accept joy into your being on every level.

Essential oil: Clary Sage

Suggested affirmation: I release all overthinking and begin to nurture myself through right thought and action.

Special application — Creating inner nourishment in your life: Skulls Safeguard can be used when you want to bring nourishment into your life, for the stomach's job is to supply nourishment at the cellular level. Just before a vacation you can treat this point to visualize how you want to nurture yourself or be nurtured on your trip. You could use the affirmation "I receive nourishment and joy as I travel and play."

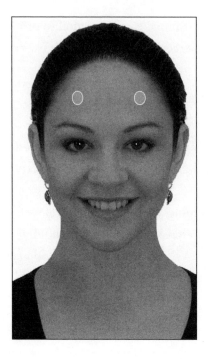

2. Yang Brightness

Meridian: Gallbladder

Meaning of name: The gallbladder meridian is a yang, or active, meridian, and is the partner of the liver. The liver controls the eyes, so it is about bringing brightness to your life and your eyes, and letting go of old thoughts and negative thinking.

Position: Above eyebrows, in the center of the forehead (position 14 along the gallbladder meridian)

Physical benefits: Brightens the eyes and improves mental clarity.

Spiritual benefits: Releases the mental congestion of old, stuck thought patterns. The gallbladder meridian influences decision making, so touching this point allows you to move forward in life and to release anger and pain.

Best time of day: 11:00 p.m.–1:00 a.m. (midnight is the peak time).

How-to: Place your thumbs or fingers right above the middle of the eyebrow at the highest point in the indentation of your forehead. Gently press upward and hold for thirty to sixty seconds.

As you press here, picture yourself gently polishing the gateway to the soul — your eyes. Relax and clear all mental tension. See yourself getting in touch with your spiritual nature, opening to new directions in your life.

Essential oil: Lavender

Suggested affirmation: I release the negativity of the past and bring health and wellness into every pore of my being.

Special application — spring renewal and planting new seeds in your life: Yang Brightness can be used as a spring pick-me-up, for the season of the gallbladder is springtime. While treating this point, you can reflect on spring renewal, using the affirmation "I replenish myself and birth myself anew, nourishing myself through this point."

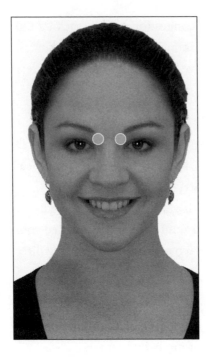

3. Eyes Bright

Meridian: Bladder

Meaning of name: This point is located in the inner corners of the eyes, so as you touch it you are stimulating the eyes and helping your vision.

Position: Insides of eye sockets, toward the bridge of the nose (position 1 on the bladder meridian, where the meridian begins)

Physical benefits: Helps the sinuses and eyes.

Spiritual benefits: Clarifies vision. Helps you begin to look at the world in a new way and focus more clearly on how to live.

Best time of day: 3:00–5:00 p.m. (4:00 p.m. is the peak time).

How-to: Place thumbs on the inside ridge of the eye sockets, close to the nose. Apply gentle pressure for one minute, taking care not to press directly on the eyes. Breathe gently and regularly.

Essential oil: None

Suggested affirmation: I see the world in a new way, with peace, calm, and inner tranquility.

Special application — releasing depression: Eyes Bright can be used to release depression and go deep inside yourself, for the bladder is connected to winter, and the associated emotion is fear. You can use the affirmation "I release fear and depression. I go deep inside myself for spiritual renewal."

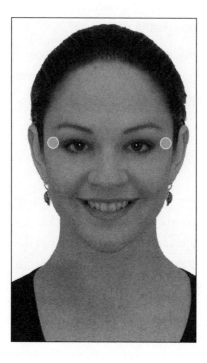

4. Pupil Bone

Meridian: Gallbladder

Meaning of name: The name of this point simply refers to its position on the face; also, it influences the pupils.

Position: Outer edges of eyebrows (position 1 on the gallbladder meridian, where the meridian begins)

Physical benefits: Increases the blood flow to the eyes and restores youthfulness to your skin.

Spiritual benefits: Enhances overall sense of well-being. The gallbladder meridian relates to decision making and the choice to bring wellness and health into your life. By stimulating this point you can choose to improve your mental and physical health and create a more positive state of mind.

Best time of day: 11:00 p.m.–1:00 a.m. (midnight is the peak time).

How-to: Place the middle fingertips below the outer edges of the eyebrows, in the hollows near the outer corners of the eyes. Press gently and hold for one minute. As you breathe in and out allow the feeling of health and wellness to spread through your body.

Essential oils: Lavender, chamomile

Suggested affirmation: As I move forward in my life, I make the decision to release negative thought patterns and have a positive state of mind and inner well-being.

Special application — releasing stress easily: Pupil Bone can be used for releasing stress, since the gallbladder meridian is related to improving your state of mind. You can use the affirmation "I now decide to release all stress and to bring calm and joy into my life."

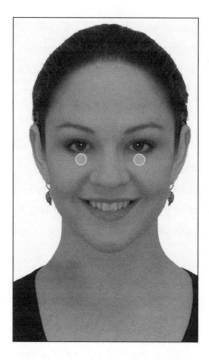

5. Receiving Cures

Meridian: Stomach

Meaning of name: This point relates to receiving the internal cures of digestion.

Position: Under the eyes (never put pressure directly on the eyeball), below the center of the eye on the ridge of the socket (position 1 on the stomach meridian, where the meridian begins)

Physical benefits: Transports nourishment to the body.

Spiritual benefits: Nurtures the spirit, feeding the inner child with love and support.

Best time of day: 7:00–9:00 a.m. (8:00 a.m. is the peak time).

How-to: Place the fingers in the indentations under the eye sockets, directly in line with the center of your pupils as you look straight ahead. Press gently and breathe softly for a count of thirty to sixty seconds.

As you work on this point, reflect on words of wisdom from your parents, or from religious or spiritual training. Words that mean a lot may include reminders to slow down, to live in the moment, to be grateful for what your have, and to appreciate yourself without comparison to others. Consider the adage, "You can't love another until you learn to love yourself." Repeating such phrases is a great way to start and end your day.

Reflect on how life has nurtured you. Feel the inner abundance and growth you have achieved in your life. Feel peace and the angelic presence of your soul. Allow this nourishment to replenish you as you go forward in your day.

Essential oils: Spruce, neroli

Suggested affirmation: I receive all that life offers to nourish me. I connect with my God-self within.

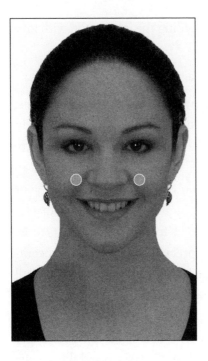

6. Welcome Fragrance

Meridian: Colon

Meaning of name: This point is located next to your sinuses, and as you breathe deeply while treating this point, you open to the fragrance of life.

Position: Cheeks, next to the nose (position 20 on the colon meridian, where the meridian ends)

Physical benefits: Improves sense of smell and eases sinus congestion.

Spiritual benefits: Welcome Fragrance helps us to release the past by allowing old memories to fade.

Best time of day: 5:00–7:00 a.m. (6:00 a.m. is the peak time).

How-to: Place the index, middle, and ring fingers next to the nose so that the ring fingers line up with the bottom of the nose. Press upward, breathing gently. Hold for a count of thirty to sixty seconds.

The colon relates to your father, the heavenly father, or the male side of your life. It helps you to release old painful feelings, such as resentment or guilt. The colon's job is to help release the past, so anything in your past relating to issues with your father, such as abuse or insecurity, can be released as you touch this point.

As you work on the colon you can release blockages of self-doubt and low self-esteem. As you release the past, begin to think about what is new and positive in your life. Refresh and feel the inner calm. Reflect on your beauty — allow this beauty to penetrate your cells.

Essential oil: Rosemary

Suggested affirmation: I release my difficulties with my father and problems regarding my spiritual essence, and I come home to my soul for guidance and protection.

Special application — releasing addictive behavior: Welcome Fragrance can be about releasing yourself from weekend indulgences or any type of addictive behavior, for the colon meridian has to do with letting go of the past. You can use the affirmation "I release all addictive behavior and bring balance into my every pore."

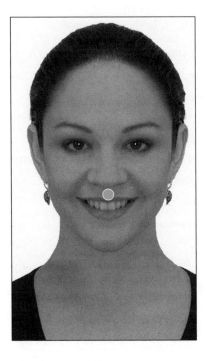

7. Middle Man

Meridian: Governor Vessel

Meaning of name: This point is located in the middle of your body, and the Governor Vessel is the most male, or yang, meridian.

Position: Upper lip (position 26 on Governor Vessel, where the meridian ends)

Physical benefits: Eases sprains, treats seizures and epilepsy, helps to bring one back to life.

Spiritual benefits: Unites masculine and feminine energies at the soul level.

Best time of day: Anytime

How-to: Place the index finger under the middle of the nose on your upper lip, midway between the top of your lip and the bottom of your nose. Push gently upward and breathe, holding for thirty to sixty seconds.

Visualize the qualities of giving and receiving. As you apply pressure here, you are helping to integrate the male and female energies in your body.

Essential oils: Ylang ylang, pine

Suggested affirmation: I bring balance and harmony into my life, giving and receiving equally.

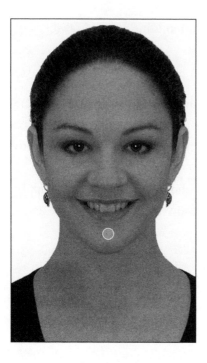

8. Receiving Fluids

Meridian: Conception Vessel

Meaning of name: This name refers to receiving inner nourishment from the internal fluids of your body.

Position: Chin (position 24 along the conception vessel)

Physical benefits: This point helps with mouth paralysis, jaw tension, and lack of coordination. By bringing fluid or secretions, it helps dryness.

Spiritual benefits: Receiving Fluids helps with anger and brings wonderful moments of inspiration and openings to your feminine nature.

Best time of day: Anytime

How-to: This point is located in the depression on the chin directly below the lower lip. Place your middle finger midway between the lower lip and the bottom of the chin. Push upward and hold for one minute.

Essential oil: Frankincense

Suggested affirmation: I flow with life and release old thoughts that inhibit my flow.

Special application — creating positive openings in your life: Receiving Fluids can be used to open yourself to abundance and invoke a positive, loving life, since the Conception Vessel is the meridian related to the feminine quality of receiving. Your affirmation could be "I am open to receiving the sweetness and goodness of the universe."

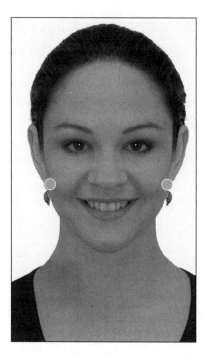

9. Lower Hinge

Meridian: Stomach

Meaning of name: This point is so named because it is located on the lower part of the jaw and is like a hinge that helps the jaw to relax.

Position: Jaw hinge, the slight indentation at the hinge of the jaw when it is open and relaxed (position 7 along the stomach meridian)

Physical benefits: This point is great for relieving temporomandibular joint (TMJ) pain, grinding of the teeth, and tightness in the jaw.

Spiritual benefits: This point helps you receive internal messages. It is located so close to the ear that it helps you to focus on what you are hearing and to filter out any negative self-talk. It provides fluidity for moving forward.

Best time of day: 7:00–9:00 a.m. (8:00 a.m. is the peak time).

How-to: This point is located two inches out from the tip of your earlobes. You can find it by opening and closing your mouth. Press the point upward and hold for one minute.

Essential oils: Peppermint, helichrysum

Suggested affirmation: I deserve to hear and receive the best that life has to give me.

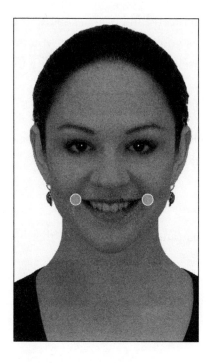

10. Stomach Granary

Meridian: Stomach

Meaning of name: This point is called the "granary" for it is where one goes to receive nourishment from food and thoughts.

Position: Mouth corners (position 4 along the stomach meridian)

Physical benefits: Helps to digest food, heals cold sores on lips, and eases toothaches.

Spiritual benefits: Begins to release the past so that you can come home to the soul.

Best time of day: 7:00–9:00 a.m. (8:00 a.m. is the peak time).

How-to: At the outside corners of the mouth, push up with the index fingers and hold for one minute, breathing deeply.

Essential oil: Rosemary

Suggested affirmation: I receive cellular regeneration and nurture my soul with divine inspiration.

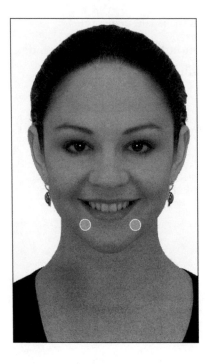

11. Mandible Wheel

Meridian: Stomach

Meaning of name: This point is located along the mandible, or lower jaw. As you touch it, it is like a wheel that influences the lower jaw and relieves stress.

Position: Chin corners, vertically halfway between tip of chin and lower lip (position 6 along the stomach meridian)

Physical benefits: Helps relieve facial twitching, tension in the jaw, and grinding of the teeth. Also calms the muscle spasms and facial contortions of Bell's palsy, a disorder of the nervous system that attacks the face.

Spiritual benefits: Helps release subconscious anger and resentments.

Best time of day: 7:00–9:00 a.m. (8:00 a.m. is the peak time).

How-to: You can find this point by placing your index fingers at the outer edges of your lips and moving straight down to the jaw line. Then move your fingertips outward along the jaw line toward your ears until you find an indentation or tender spot. Your fingertips should end on a position vertically midway between your chin and lower lip. Press and hold for one minute.

Essential oil: Lavender

Suggested affirmation: I release old fears and focus on self-love and nourishment.

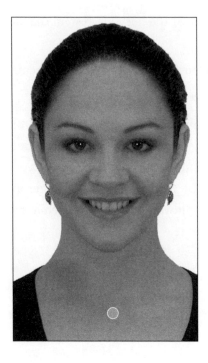

12. Angel Spring

Meridian: Conception Vessel

Meaning of name: When you touch this point, you connect with your angelic essence and your wellspring of pure love and speech.

Position: Base of throat (position 23 along the Conception Vessel)

Physical benefits: Helps to clear speech, ease coughing, and relieve throat inflammation. Helps stimulate the thymus.

Spiritual benefits: Helps you to speak the truth. This point helps open you to your divine nature. It connects you with your inner spirituality.

As you breathe with this point, you connect with the divine truth of who you are at your core.

Best time of day: First thing in the morning, or anytime

How-to: You locate this point by moving a finger directly down the middle of your throat to the Adam's apple. You hold this point for one minute, then release, touching it gently and with love. Continue breathing as you apply pressure to this area.

Essential oil: Clary sage

Suggested affirmation: I speak my truth with joy as I move into the inner core of my being.

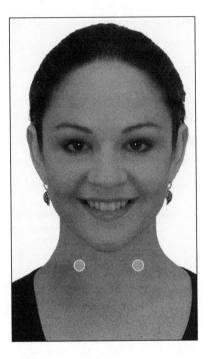

13. Greeting Welcome

Meridian: Stomach

Meaning of name: This point is so named because it will help you greet the day with joy and self-love.

Position: Neck (position 9 along the stomach meridian)

Physical benefits: Regulates energy and blood, clears throat constrictions. This point stimulates the thymus and thus strengthens your immune system.

Spiritual benefits: Encourages awakening, openness, and self-care. When you feel "fed up" or you "have had it up to here," touching this point helps leave behind old resentments and awakens you to your inner clarity. Greeting Welcome (also called Window of Sky) opens you to your spiritual essence.

Best time of day: 7:00–9:00 a.m. (8:00 a.m. is the peak time).

How-to: Relax with your hands in your lap for a few seconds. With your index and middle fingers, gently tap your chin for a few seconds; then tap halfway down your neck. Gently place your fingers at either side of the windpipe and press just enough to feel the pressure. Tap your fingers up and down the neck.

As you apply gentle pressure here, reflect on past resentments and times you have taken care of others at the expense of yourself. With each exhale, release those emotions, and with each inhale breathe in love toward others and yourself.

Essential oil: Frankincense

Suggested affirmation: I connect with my spiritual essence and live my truth with dignity.

AS YOU CONCLUDE YOUR ACUPRESSURE FACELIFT, take a moment to sense how you feel. Move into the rest of your day with grace.

CHAPTER FIVE

Acupressure Treatments for Common Maladies That Show in the Face

It's no wonder that friends and family members sometimes say, "You don't look well today." Illness, pain, and disease are all reflected in our faces — not simply in our expressions, but also in the coloring and appearance of our skin.

In the ancient traditions of Chinese medicine, healers have always used the patient's face to diagnose disease and to assess how well or poorly the body's major organs are functioning. Today the professional acupuncture or acupressure practitioner will spend time with you not only discussing your symptoms but also looking at your face, studying the visible clues as to what is going on inside your body.

You, too, are capable of assessing the functioning of your body's organs. You simply have to know what to look for. The following information will help you find the link between your facial indicators and problems or potential problems in your organic system. Once you know these things, you can apply the appropriate acupressure treatment to release discordant energy, rebalance your system, and begin to heal in body, mind, and spirit. As you regenerate and heal inside, your face will reflect the healthy path you have chosen for yourself.

This section addresses common conditions in the body that can be detected in the face. These conditions — ranging from dizziness to diarrhea — can be successfully treated with acupressure. For each one, I offer simple acupressure exercises to bring you relief, bolstering body and spirit.

As you know, many of the meridians begin and end on the face and go through the different layers of the skin as well as through the organs. You can tell how healthy your organs are by observing the colors on your face. For example, if you see a greenish or yellowish tinge on the outer edge of the eye, it may signal that your digestive tract needs help; green circulates to the liver, and the liver controls the eyes, while yellow circulates to the spleen or stomach. On the other hand, if you have blue-black circles under your eyes, this could indicate a kidney or bladder imbalance.

As you do the exercises, breathe slowly, inhaling a sense of calm and well-being and exhaling anything you would like to release — problems, trauma, fear, worry, and old, unneeded emotions that have stopped you from expressing yourself. Focus your mind on sustaining calm, and imagine health for mind, body, and spirit. Feel the flow of energy among the different points stimulated in each exercise.

Minor Stomach Cramps and Intestinal Gas

Facial indicator: Yellow tinges at sides of face
Affected organs: Stomach, spleen
Emotional pattern: Overthinking, anxiety
Acupressure points: Rib cage, groin, inner thighs
Best time of day: 8:00 a.m., the peak time of the stomach

How-to:

1. While sitting in a chair with your back straight, cup the fingers of both hands over the sides of your rib cage. Clasp firmly, breathe deeply several times, and hold the position for three minutes.

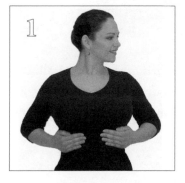

2. Move your fingers down to press on both sides of your groin. Hold for three minutes. This releases tension in the groin and helps the colon to relax.

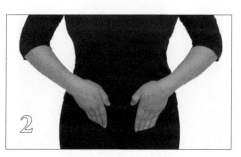

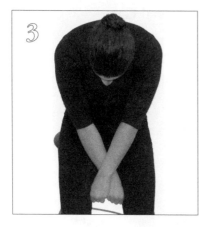

3. Sitting in a chair, squeeze your hands into fists, then cross your arms at the waist and place your fists between your inner thighs, about three inches above your knees. Press your fists into your thighs as firmly as possible and hold for three minutes. As you press on these points, you are releasing stress in the legs, which, both practically and symbolically, helps you to move forward.

Suggested affirmations: I allow life to flow through me effortlessly. I live in divine harmony. I live in the moment. I love myself. I receive nourishment of my inner being through my connection to the Divine.

More Severe Stomach Cramps

Facial indicator: Crow's feet
Affected organs: Stomach, spleen
Emotional pattern: Worry, stress
Acupressure points: Biceps, rib cage, inner thighs
Best time of day: 8:00 a.m., the peak time of the stomach

How-to:

1. Cross the arms over the chest with each hand resting on the opposite arm. Press the thumbs into the biceps and gently hold for three minutes.

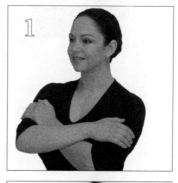

2. While sitting in a chair with your back straight, cup the fingers of both hands over the sides of the rib cage. Clasp firmly, breathe deeply several times, and hold the position for three minutes.

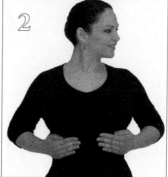

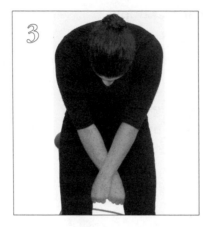

3. Sitting in a chair, squeeze your hands into fists, then cross your arms at the waist and place your fists between your inner thighs, about three inches above your knees. Press your fists into your thighs as firmly as possible and hold for three minutes.

Suggested affirmations: I let go of the need to control. I open to receive all of the inner nourishment from my soul.

Low Energy, Tension, Stiffness, and Stress (Especially in the Back)

Facial indicator: Bluish circles, darkened area of the eyes

Affected organs: Bladder, kidneys

Emotional pattern: Feeling stuck in life, fear

Acupressure points: Shoulders, upper back, central lower back, base of spine

Best time of day: 4:00 p.m., the peak time of the bladder meridian, which goes down the back alongside the spine

How-to:

1. Sitting in a chair with your back straight, rest your hands on your shoulders. Depending on which is more comfortable, you may either cross your arms in front of you and place each hand on the opposite shoulder, or you may place your right hand on your right shoulder and your left hand on your left 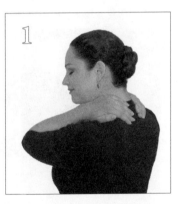 shoulder (as shown in the photograph). With your fingers, apply gentle pressure to your upper back. Breathe deeply in and out. Hold for three minutes.

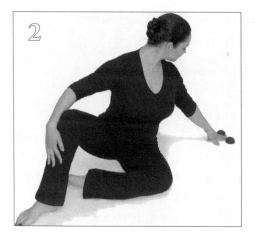

2. Sit on the floor with your knees bent. Place two Helping Hands on the floor behind you, a few inches apart. Lie down, positioning the Helping Hands under the middle of each shoulder blade. Place both fists, knuckles up, on the underside of your waist, close to your spine. Relax and lie in this position for three minutes. These points near the lower spine focus on releasing energy from the kidneys.

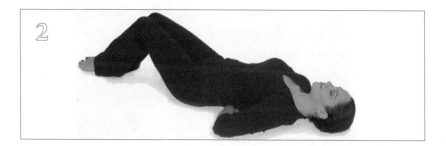

3. Still lying down with the Helping Hands under your shoulder blades, place both hands, palms down, under your buttocks at the level of your hips. Hold for three minutes. With your hands in this position, you may feel the coccyx (a point at the base of the

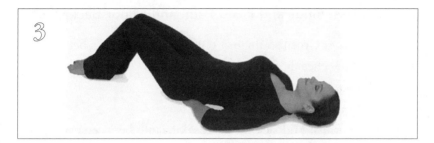

spine), called Long and Strong in Chinese medicine, starting to relax. Notice a sense of rejuvenation coming into your spinal cord, and relax at all levels of your being.

When you work on the bladder and kidneys, you rejuvenate the spinal column. In addition, the bladder meridian runs through every organ in the body. Thus, working in this position gives every cell, every organ, and every tissue the energy to rejuvenate itself.

Suggested affirmations: I release the past and anything that is holding me back in my life.

Dizziness, Sinus and Head Pain, and Minor Backache

Facial indicator: Greenish tinge at either side of the face between the
eyes and the cheekbones

Affected organs: Liver, gallbladder

Emotional pattern: Feeling stuck in life, fear

Acupressure points: Midback, neck, base of skull, between eyes, pubic
bone

Best time of day: Midnight, the peak time of the gallbladder; however,
since you're likely to be sleeping at that time, perform these exercises as late in the evening as possible

How-to:

1. Lie on your back and place a Helping Hand under your waist,
at the point in the midback called Gate of Life, which correlates

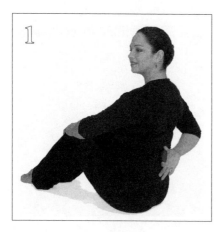

to the kidneys or adrenals. This
point will strengthen your back,
for the kidneys control the
back. As you lie for three minutes with gentle pressure
on this point, visualize inner
strength coming into your
essence. Keep the Helping
Hand under your back for the
remainder of the exercises in
this sequence.

2. Place your left hand under your neck and press gently. Relax and hold for three minutes.

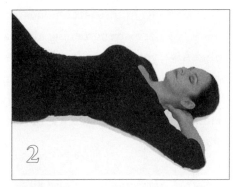

3. Place your hands on the indentation on either side of the base of your skull and press gently. Hold for three minutes.

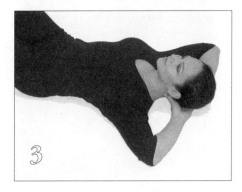

4. Use your right thumb to press on the indentation between your eyes at the top of your nose. At the same time, press on your pubic bone with your left hand. Hold for three minutes. (You may have your right leg bent, as in the photograph, or extended.)

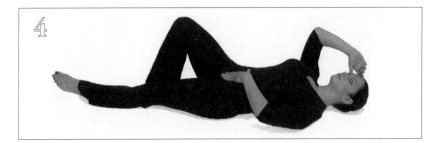

The results of these techniques are many. With the first three exercises, you are strengthening the back and increasing your well-being. Also, you are relaxing the entire spinal column, renewing your inner stability and groundedness, and connecting with spiritual essence and both heavenly and earthly energy. And with the fourth technique, you will feel a sense of relaxation in the sinuses and pubic bone.

Suggested affirmations: I release all fear. I choose to live my life in excitement and joy.

Dizziness, Tired Eyes, and Pressure at the Base of the Skull

Facial indicator: Vertical lines between the brows
Affected organs: Liver, eyes
Emotional pattern: Anger and the inability to express it
Acupressure points: Brow bone, lower back, base of skull
Best time of day: From 1:00 to 3:00 a.m., the peak time of the liver; however, since you're likely to be sleeping at that time, perform these exercises as late in the evening as possible

How-to:

1. Place your thumbs on the bone directly below your eyebrows at the inside curve of the bridge of the nose. Press gently upward, taking care not to put pressure directly on the eyes, and hold for three minutes.

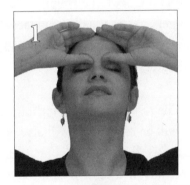

2. Place a Helping Hand under the spine at the waistline and lie back on it. Rest there for three minutes.

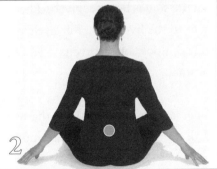

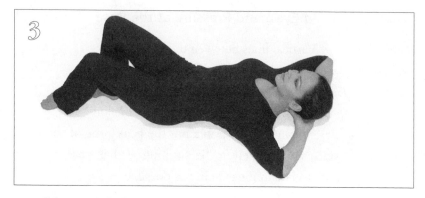

3. Still lying with the Helping Hand under your back, lace your fingers together and then place them under the base of your skull. Press your hands into both sides of the skull. Hold for three minutes.

The result of the first technique is that sinus pressure and congestion will be relieved. It will also bring relaxation to the eyes and help you to see the world in a new way. You will experience a stronger, more enlivened sense of spiritual essence, and you will have a feeling that the soul is being revived. The second technique brings replenishment to the liver. The third releases the eyes and begins to brighten your outlook and rejuvenate you on all levels: physical, mental, and spiritual.

Suggested affirmations: I see the world in a new way. I am connected to all things with love and harmony. Love flows through me.

Poor Circulation, High or Low Blood Pressure, Angina, or Irregular Heartbeats

Facial indicator: Red/flushed cheeks

Affected organs: Heart, pericardium

Emotional pattern: Lack of joy, emotional disheartenment, disinterest in life

Acupressure points: Calves

Best time of day: Noon, the peak time of the heart

How-to:

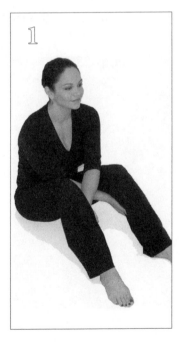

1. Seated with your back straight, plant your feet firmly on the ground. At the bottom of each foot there is a point called Bubbling Spring, which opens the body to new circulation, new ways to walk on the earth; your legs are very important in helping you move forward in a new direction. Spread your knees apart to about shoulder width and lean forward. Cross your arms in front of you, placing your right palm on your left calf and your left palm on your right calf. Press gently and hold for three minutes.

2. Now, reverse the cross of the arms; whichever arm was on top now crosses to the bottom. Again place each palm on the opposite calf. Press gently and hold for an additional three minutes.

This technique will aid the cardiovascular system, especially the heart and its partner, the pericardium. This helps to regulate the circulatory system. As a result, you may become very warm.

Suggested affirmations: I now circulate self-love to every cell of my being. I live in love, and with joy I release all negativity. I release self-doubt and bring in self-assurance.

Menstrual Problems and Menopausal Symptoms

Facial indicator: Red, flushed cheeks

Affected organ: Liver

Emotional pattern: Irritability, frequent crying

Acupressure points: Upper back, biceps, base of skull, rib cage, tailbone, pubic bone

Best time of day: From 1:00 to 3:00 a.m., the peak time of the liver; however, since you're likely to be sleeping at that time, perform these exercises as late in the evening as possible

How-to:

1. Sitting on the floor, place a Helping Hand on the floor behind you. Lie on your back, positioning the Helping Hand under your spine between the shoulder blades. Cross your arms comfortably over your chest and press your thumbs into your biceps. Hold for three minutes.

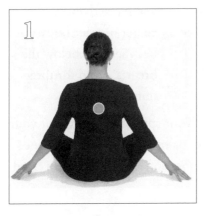
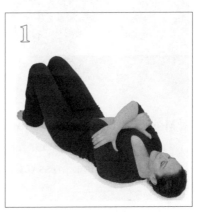

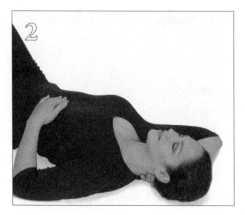

2. Still lying with the Helping Hand between your shoulder blades, move your right hand to the center of the base of your skull and place your left hand on the base of your breast-bone. Hold for three minutes.

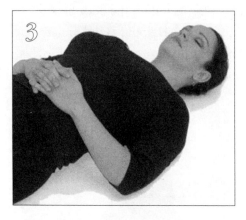

3. Still lying with the Helping Hand between your shoulder blades, gently interlace your fingers, with fingertips down, and place them on the center of your body, between and below the breasts. Hold for three minutes.

4. Move the Helping Hand lower on your spine, to the level of your waistline, and place your left hand, palm up, under the tailbone. At the same time, press on your pubic bone with your right hand.

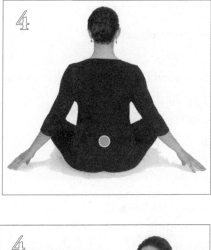

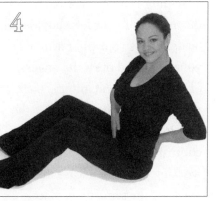

Hold for three minutes. (The second photo shows the correct hand placement, but you should remain lying down while you perform the exercise.)

The liver is often responsible for hormonal problems. You can expect many rewards when you do these exercises. During the first one, as the tension and heat start to leave the body, you will experience total relaxation and inner calm in every cell. When you perform the second one, you will feel the body begin to release tension in the jaw and upper back. With the third technique, you are relaxing the diaphragm, enabling digestion, and relieving mental tension and stress. The fourth will balance masculine and feminine energies in the body, so that you feel more at ease and balanced.

Suggested affirmation: My life flows easily with joy.

Diarrhea and Excess Stomach Acid

Facial indicator: Horizontal lines on the forehead
Affected organs: Colon, stomach
Emotional pattern: Holding on; unresolved issues with father; excessive behaviors, such as "running off at the mouth"
Acupressure points: Shoulder, buttocks, tailbone
Best time of day: 6:00 a.m., the peak time of the colon

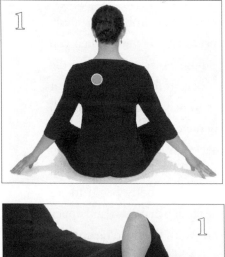

How-to:

1. Begin by lying on your back with a Helping Hand positioned under the middle of your left shoulder blade. Cross your right arm over your chest and press the fingers of your right hand into the back of your left shoulder, just above the shoulder blade. The need for control resides in this area, and working here can release this need. At the same time, place your left hand, palm down, under your left buttock. Hold for three minutes.

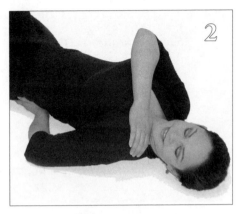

2. Then, keeping your right hand in the same position, move your left hand so that your fingertips are pressing into the left side of your tailbone. Hold for three minutes.

Important note: Never reverse the order of the steps in this routine. Doing so can upset the digestive tract.

On the spiritual level, this technique will help reestablish your connection to the areas of your life that have gotten out of control. You will begin restoring the natural balance of your system in all aspects of life. Your body, mind, and spirit will no longer be beyond your control.

Suggested affirmations: I stay in balance. I do not overextend. With the Creator's help, I remain in control.

Constipation and Colitis

Facial indicator: Vertical lines from the sides of the nose to the sides of the mouth

Affected organ: Colon

Emotional pattern: Holding on and working against the natural flow of life

Acupressure points: Upper back, inner thigh, buttocks

Best time of day: 6:00 a.m., the peak time of the colon

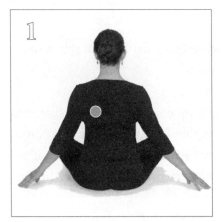

How-to:

1. Lie on your back, positioning a Helping Hand under your left shoulder blade. Place your right foot on your left knee. Press your left hand into your right inner thigh and hold this position for three minutes.

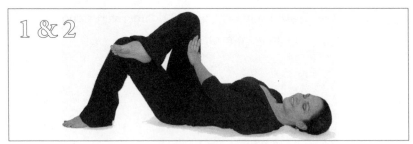

2. Still lying with the Helping Hand under your back and your left hand on your right thigh, make a fist with your right hand and place it under your right buttock. Hold for three minutes. As you work with this point, you will begin to experience calm and peace of mind.

Important note: As with the previous sequence, never reverse the order of the steps in this routine. Doing so can upset the digestive tract.

The result of this technique is that your bowels will flow smoothly, and you will easily be able to let go of negative thoughts.

Suggested affirmations: I flow with life effortlessly. I relax and allow all the good of the universe to come to me.

CHAPTER SIX

Nutrition for Healthy Skin and a Healthy Body

The food we eat is extremely important to our physical, mental, and spiritual health and to longevity. When we consume too much acid, fat, or alcohol, our health suffers. As one system is upset, other processes in the body are affected, and the entire balance can be thrown off. Abusive patterns relating to food, such as bingeing, can lead to a buildup of toxins, a compromised immune system, bad digestion, headaches, back pain, and other, more serious problems. Your body will tell you what it needs. You just have to understand the signals and respond in a way that eliminates negative energy and removes toxins from your system, replacing them with the positive energy of nourishing foods. Whenever possible, eats fresh fruits and vegetables that are grown locally and organically (that is, without synthetic pesticides or herbicides), for these have the purest energy of all. Similarly, choose meats that are organic and free-range and fish that is wild or sustainably farmed.

Guidelines for Healthy Eating from the Chinese Tradition

Chinese medicine offers numerous guidelines for maintaining a healthy diet. They are as follows:

- Eat in moderation. This is one of the secrets of longevity. Too much food injures the stomach and spleen and causes many ills, including indigestion, urinary and bowel imbalances, disturbed sleep patterns, and obesity. You should stop eating just before feeling completely full and should always eat lightly at night so the body can completely digest the day's food. This allows the stomach to do its job properly.

- Eat at regular intervals. This allows the body to function with a regular rhythm. Eating moderate amounts every few hours, rather than eating only one or two large meals a day, aids in digestion.

- Eat lightly one day a week to give the stomach, spleen, and pancreas a rest.

- Eat warm, nurturing foods, for they contribute to healthy digestion (see the section on page 90 on food categories).

- Avoid excessively hot or cold foods. Too much hot food will damage the heart. Too much cold food will damage the spleen and digestive tract.

- Eat a balanced combination of the basic flavors — sweet, sour, bitter, salty, and pungent. Too much sweet will damage the spleen; too much sour will damage the liver; too much bitter will damage the heart and small intestine; too much salt will damage the kidneys; too much pungent (curries, for example) will damage the colon.

- Limit your intake of dairy (i.e., foods containing cheese or milk), which can clog your spleen, liver, and lungs and produce puffiness in your face and phlegm in your system.

- Eat yellow- or orange-colored foods to aid digestion, for the yellow color relates to the spleen. These foods, such as sweet potato and squash, aid digestion. (You will also aid digestion when you work on the facial points under your eyes.)

- Eat steamed green leafy vegetables and room-temperature salads, for they aid the liver in detoxification.

- Eat small amounts of meat to nurture the bone marrow and keep the blood healthy. Deficiencies in the blood can lead to low energy, anxiety, and pale skin.

- To treat constipation, start the day by drinking a cup of hot water and lemon juice to help cleanse the liver.

- Always eat with a positive attitude. Having negative conversations, reading the newspaper, working at a computer, or watching TV while eating can upset the digestive tract. Thinking positive thoughts, on the other hand, nourishes the soul while the meal is nourishing the body.

- Always eat in a relaxed environment. Make sure you take your time; do not eat on the run, for doing so is a shock to your colon and stomach, and the stress can cause worry lines around the mouth. Never eat when you're upset; food taken in at this time can act like a poison, disturbing the ascent and descent of chi and resulting in stagnation.

- When you sit down to eat a meal, first offer a prayer to bless your food; when you do that, you are showing appreciation for life.

- While eating, focus on your digestion.

- Eat slowly and chew thoroughly; this will promote healthy digestion and the absorption of enzymes.

- Eat natural foods that are prepared with love.

- Take a leisurely walk after eating, for this aids digestion by stimulating the flow of chi and the blood. The Chinese say that if a person walks one hundred paces after a meal, he or she may live ninety-nine years.

- Avoid watching television right after eating. Instead, listen to soft music, which will aid digestion.

Food Categories: Hot, Warm, Cool, Cold, and Neutral

The Chinese classify foods into five categories — hot, warm, cool, cold, and neutral. These classifications refer to the effects the foods have on the body when eaten, not to the temperatures of the foods themselves. Here is a list of common foods that fit into each category:

Hot	Warm	Cool	Cold	Neutral
butter	asparagus	apple	bamboo shoot	almonds
cardamom	beef	avocado	banana	apricot
chilies	chicken	barley	bean sprout	cabbage
chocolate	coconut	broccoli	cauliflower	carrot
cinnamon	coffee	celery	clams	corn
cottonseed oil	coriander	cucumber	crab	duck
curry	date	eggplant	grapefruit	egg
ginger, dried	fennel	mango	green tea	grapes
lamb	garlic	marjoram	hops	honey
onion	ginger, fresh	mung bean	ice cream	milk
peanut butter	ginseng	mushroom, button	kelp/seaweed	mushroom, shiitake
pepper, black or white	green onion	orange	lettuce	olives
pepper, red or green	guava	pear	mussels	oysters
smoked fish	ham	peppermint	persimmon	papaya
soybean oil	leek	pineapple	salt	peanuts
trout	oats	radish	tofu/bean curd	plum
whiskey	peach	sesame oil	tomato	pork
	shrimp	spinach	water chestnut	potato
	squash, summer and winter	strawberry	watermelon	rice
	sugar, brown	turnip	yogurt	salmon
	vinegar	wheat		sugar, white
	walnuts			sweet potato
	wine			

Warm foods are the most nurturing and nourishing. They dispel cold energy and increase the circulation of chi, so you should try to eat as many of them as possible. However, you should balance these with cool and cold foods. Also, practitioners of Chinese medicine believe that cool foods should be eaten in warm weather, and warm foods should be eaten when the weather turns cold.

Some conditions in the body indicate an imbalance of warm and cool. For example, a fever or sore throat is an indication that the body is holding too much heat, while cold hands and feet show that the body is running cold. These conditions can be corrected by consuming the appropriate warm or cool foods.

To cool the body, you should consume cooling foods such as mint, watermelon, or green tea. To warm the body, eat warm foods such as soups, herbs, and red Chinese dates (called *du ʒao*; available at Asian markets). Keep in mind that certain cold or cool foods can be made warm with additives; for example, tofu and soy products — generally considered cold foods — can be warmed with garlic or ginger.

In cooking food, steaming brings cool properties to foods, while stir-frying adds heat.

What the Hands and Feet Say

Practitioners of Chinese medicine see the hands as microcosms of the entire body, so they pay particular attention to the hands as a diagnostic indicator of what is occurring elsewhere in the body. The following chart shows some common conditions of the hands, what those conditions indicate, and possible remedies.

Condition of Hands	Indication	Remedy Options
Hot, dry, scaly, red	Excessive internal heat	Mint tea, green tea, apple juice, grape juice, orange peel tea
Cold, pale	Excessive internal cold	Dong quai (a Chinese herb), Chinese licorice root (fresh or dried)
Clammy	Too much fat in the diet; excessive moisture, dampness	Peony tea, Chinese red dates, cinnamon
Ridges on fingernails	Liver imbalance	Honey, celery, basil, fennel, oats, kudzu root, flax
Brittle, flaky nails	Liver imbalance	Blueperium (a Chinese herb)

When you take the time to massage your hands with a natural lotion, such as one containing jojoba, you are helping to balance and relax your entire system.

Working with the hands also contributes to health in the eyes, face, and back. The feet, too, are seen as indicators of the health elsewhere in the body. For example, you can work with your feet and toes to balance the sinuses, help circulation, and release stagnant chi. To stimulate your internal organs, you can roll your feet back and forth over a tennis ball or any small ball.

Guidelines for Consuming Liquids

Along with eating properly, it is also important to keep yourself hydrated. You should drink at least eight glasses of water every day. It is best to not drink liquids during meals; instead, liquids should be taken a half hour after meals to aid digestion. They should be at room temperature, since your body is 98° and cold water will shock your system. From the perspective of Chinese medicine, ice water will slow digestion. It is a good idea, though, to drink hot water with lemon, especially first thing in the morning.

The Chinese keep a keen eye on the liquids they consume, because they know that too much liquid can cause a painful illness called *dampness*, a condition wherein liquid collects in the body and becomes stagnant. Dampness blocks the flow of chi and can hamper functioning of the spleen and kidneys. We experience dampness as lethargy, poor circulation, puffy eyes, and bloating. When it occurs, it is difficult to displace. A nonspicy diet with cooked vegetables and rice (the Chinese consider rice the most nurturing grain) helps remove dampness. Clear soups also can decrease it and other conditions clogging your system.

Alcohol is hot, and consuming too much can injure the blood and cause a decline of chi. However, one glass of red wine with a meal can aid circulation.

Herbal Teas

Teas have been an important part of Chinese culture since ancient times and have been used for millennia to replenish, restore, and rejuvenate. Medicinal herbal teas are a cornerstone of Chinese medicine. They can help the body in a variety of ways: they can aid digestion, stimulate metabolism, balance hormones, improve the immune system, purify the blood, and regulate blood pressure. A huge variety of packaged herbal teas are available at natural food stores, but another option is to purchase fresh herbs and make herbal teas yourself.

To do so, place the herbs in a pot containing enough water to cover the herbs by about an inch and a half. If possible, use spring water or other purified drinking water. Let the herbs soak in the water for about fifteen minutes before turning on the heat. Bring the water to a rolling boil and then turn the heat down to a low simmer.

Different types of herbs vary greatly in the amount of time they should steep, or simmer, but here are some guidelines:

- Barks, such as cinnamon or sassafras: 20 minutes

- Hard roots, such as comfrey or burdock: 20 minutes

- Soft roots, such as licorice or marshmallow: 10 to 15 minutes

- Flowers, such as hibiscus or chamomile: 10 to 20 minutes

- Seeds, such as fennel: 5 to 10 minutes

- Berries, such as hawthorn or juniper: 5 to 10 minutes

The exception to these instructions are leaves, such as peppermint or nettle, which should never be boiled or simmered; instead, boil only the water, then turn off the heat, add the leaves, and steep for 20 minutes.

Digestion and Detoxification

According to Chinese medicine, colon health is an important element of overall well-being and is critical to longevity; therefore, you must try to keep the digestive tract flowing smoothly. To maximize the health of your digestive tract and colon, you should eliminate first thing in the morning, between five o'clock and seven o'clock. Then, before eating, you can drink warm water with lemon juice to stimulate digestion. This drink will also cleanse the liver. Below is a list of foods that promote healthy digestion and detoxification.

If you suffer from diarrhea or loose bowel movements, your body is probably holding toxins in the intestinal tract, possibly from eating contaminated food or drink — or the emotional body may be suffering an upset. In this state, you should avoid consuming oils, fats, leafy vegetables, and milk products. Too much dairy causes phlegm in the intestinal tract and makes the body sluggish.

Foods for Healthy Digestion	Foods for Detoxification
apple	apple
bok choy	broccoli
chicken	cashews
date	chicken
fennel seed	pork
fish	raisins
papaya	snow pea
spinach	spinach
tofu or tempeh	squash
yam	tofu or tempeh

To remove toxins from the intestines and help with diarrhea, boil a cup of rice, either brown or white, in four cups of water for ten to fifteen minutes. Then strain the rice and drink the remaining water. You may eat or discard the rice.

Chinese licorice tea also helps remove toxins from the system. Boil four cups of water in a glass pan or saucepan. Add several pieces of Chinese licorice root (available in Asian markets or natural food stores). Return to a boil and simmer for twenty minutes or until the liquid is reduced by half. Strain. You may add honey to suit your taste.

Eating for the Skin

The following foods are especially nurturing for the skin. You may eat them separately or in combination with other foods.

- Fruits, especially avocado, blackberries, cherries, lemon, dates, and cantaloupe

- Vegetables, especially broccoli, ginger, seaweed (for its high mineral content), sweet potato, and orange-colored squash

- Grains such as brown rice, sesame seeds, and sunflower seeds

- Protein, including organic free-range chicken and fish such as cod, haddock, scrod, flounder, salmon, and whitefish

Avoid alcohol, fried foods, and dairy products. These clog your pores and can cause oiliness in the skin.

Dietary Recommendations for Different Skin Types

In chapter 2 we learned about different skin types and how to treat them. Along with the techniques described there, you can support your skin by eating well. Below I outline what kinds of foods you should eat for your skin type.

Normal Skin

Those with normal skin should avoid eating fried foods or eating while under stress, for this turns the body acidic, which is toxic. Traditionally, Chinese women eat walnuts and rice for breakfast, for these foods have natural oils that lubricate without clogging the skin. They also drink mint tea each day or put mint on their skin to cool the blood and to help the body withstand heat and maintain its natural balance.

If you have normal skin, you can keep it healthy by eating green leafy vegetables, whole grains, and squash. An excellent combination for normal skin is salmon and asparagus — these foods together are very neutral for normal skin, help oxygenate the body, bolster the digestive tract and circulation, and help moisturize the lungs. They will also promote a dewy, youthful look. Chicken and cod are other good protein choices for normal skin.

The following herbal teas are also great for those with normal skin: lavender, chamomile, fennel, comfrey, and calendula.

Dry Skin

If your skin is very dry, it's important to add oil to your diet, possibly by eating avocado once or twice a week. Aduki beans, papaya, black sesame seeds, ginger, royal jelly, and gelatin will increase the elasticity of your entire system. Avoid grapefruit, radishes, vinegar, and hard liquor; these will aggravate your condition. Clear-broth soups will also help when you have dry skin.

Teas that nourish dry skin include slippery elm, which lubricates the skin and aids digestion, ginseng tea, and Throat Coat tea, an herbal tea blend made by Traditional Medicinals and available at natural food stores.

Oily Skin

For those with oily skin, the goal is to eat more cooling foods, such as carrot, mint, peas, pear, spinach, and watermelon. Cold cucumber soup will help cool your system, and I have provided a recipe for it on the next page.

If you have oily skin, be sure to drink plenty of water. Avoid hot, spicy foods such as chili peppers, as well as fried foods and alcohol, for these will dilate your blood vessels. Avoid fats and sweets. Avoid alcohol-based skin-cleansing and -toning products.

Herbs and teas that will help balance oily skin include chamomile, which helps relax the nervous system; chrysanthemum, a pick-me-up that helps cool your system when you feel hot; peppermint, which is wonderful for digestion and calms upset stomachs; and lemongrass.

Recipe: Cucumber Soup

This soup will help balance oily skin and will help relieve rashes or skin irritation.

2 cucumbers, peeled, seeded, and chopped
2 garlic cloves, peeled and chopped
1 small onion, peeled and quartered
1 tsp. fresh lemon juice
a few pieces of ice

Place half of the cucumber and the garlic, onion, and ice in a blender and process until smooth. Then add the remaining cucumber and the lemon juice. Stir. Serve in chilled soup bowls.

For acne-prone skin, licorice and yarrow teas are cooling and help to dispel the heat causing the acne.

Combination Skin

For combination skin, foods such as corn, celery, lettuce, spinach, and fish help balance the skin as well as aid in digestion and help replenish the stomach, spleen, lungs, and colon. Also, parsley will help balance the pH of the skin.

Sensitive Skin

Sensitive skin indicates that your colon may be clogged, so you need to purify your skin and help your body to perspire. Eat dishes containing ginger or pepper, for these spices will open your pores and help you to perspire.

If you have brown spots on your skin, called liver spots, blend one papaya (chopped into pieces) with the juice of one lemon and one tablespoon of raw honey. Rub the mixture on your skin and leave it for five minutes. Rinse and dry your skin gently.

Vitamins and Minerals for the Skin and Body

In an ideal world, we would get all the nutrients we need from the foods we eat. However, sometimes that's not possible, so it's important to supplement the diet with vitamins, minerals, and herbs. A list of the vitamins that tend to be lacking in the Western diet follows.

- Vitamin A is necessary for good eyesight. Also, it strengthens the tissue of the lungs, intestines, and mucus membranes, which helps protect the skin from sun damage and promotes flexibility of the joints. You should not take more than 15,000 IU (international units) per day, for an excess of vitamin A can be toxic to the body.

- Vitamin C is an antioxidant, and antioxidants are believed to help protect against cancer. Vitamin C is also integral to collagen formation in the skin and cartilage and helps prevent the breakage of capillary walls. You can get vitamin C from citrus fruits, bell peppers, and dark green leafy vegetables. Limit your intake of vitamin C to 500 to 1,000 milligrams per day; more than this can cause diarrhea.

- Vitamin D is produced in the skin through the absorption of sunlight. It helps the body to absorb calcium, which is necessary for bone development. Lack of vitamin D can cause osteoporosis. Aside from spending time in the sun, you can get vitamin D from fish oils, fortified milk, and egg yolks.

- Vitamin E is another antioxidant, and it protects the tissues of the body. Avocados, wheat germ, and green leafy vegetables are good sources of vitamin E.

- Vitamin K facilitates blood coagulation and is found in spinach and broccoli.

Additionally, your body requires certain minerals:

- Calcium to strengthen teeth and bones.

- Magnesium to synthesize protein and to protect the heart.

- Potassium to balance the body's pH, increase energy, and improve muscular movement.

- Sodium to regulate water levels and to transport minerals through the cell membranes.

What the Tongue Says

Practitioners of Chinese medicine view the tongue as an important diagnostic tool. In an examination, they will look closely at the tongue to get information about your diet and overall health. A healthy tongue should be pink and moist with a thin clear or white coat. Observing your own tongue can give you a sense of what improvements you could make in your diet.

- If your tongue is red or has red marks, this indicates too much heat in the body. To correct this, you can eat more cooling foods, such as cucumber and the other cool and cold foods listed on page 91.

- If your tongue is pale, this indicates you should eat more warming foods.

- If you have teeth marks on the outer edges of your tongue, this indicates poor digestion. Eat yellow or orange vegetables, such as squash and sweet potato.

A Healthy Diet for a Healthy Day

Here is a suggested plan for your daily diet:

1. Begin the day by looking in the mirror and seeing that you are the face of God.

2. Before eating, drink an eight-ounce glass of hot water with the juice of half a lemon.

3. Eat a breakfast that consists of some sort of warm food or cereal, for this aids digestion.

4. At midmorning, eat an apple or other fruit.

5. Eat warm foods for lunch, such as soup, steamed fish, and steamed vegetables.

6. Eat a light dinner — a warm soup would be perfect.

IN ADDITION TO THE DIETARY GUIDELINES included here, the Chinese advocate adjusting the diet according to the seasonal cycle. In the next chapter we'll learn how to eat — and live — in tune with the seasons.

CHAPTER SEVEN

Living in Harmony
with the Seasons

Farmers — those who plant, nurture, and harvest crops and then allow the ground to lie fallow for a period of rest — know well the significance of the seasons. Practitioners of the principles of Chinese medicine also honor the seasons, understanding that a healthy life is one that follows the seasonal cycle of nature. As we learn about the ebb and flow of the seasons and their intent for us, we learn to tune in to our own natural rhythms and adjust our lifestyles in accordance with them.

Each season deals with rejuvenation in a specific context. Springtime is the season for new ideas, a time for laying both short- and long-term foundations. Summer is the season to nourish those ideas and watch them take root and grow. Indian summer, which the Chinese view as a season unto itself, is a time to prepare for the rest and reflection to come in the seasons that follow. Fall is the harvest season, a time for gathering up thoughts and ideas — a time to begin putting our lives in order. Winter is the time to go within, to be quiet in preparation for the new beginning in the next sequence of seasons. Also, each season governs two meridians (except summer, which governs four) and the corresponding organs, as explained in the description of each season that follows.

Spring: March 21 to June 20

Spring is the season for recognizing life as a beautiful pathway filled with new opportunities, a time for spiritual regeneration and finding peace of mind. It is a time to plan ahead, to consider goals and dreams, and to plant new ideas.

The liver and gallbladder are the meridians related to springtime. There are forty-four points along the gallbladder meridian; it starts by the outer corner of the eye, goes over the top of the head, down the side of the body, and ends on the fourth toe. The liver meridian has fourteen points. It begins on the inside of the big toe and runs up the inside of the leg and ends under the rib cage.

The gallbladder rules decision making, while the liver is associated with the actions that decisions require — making plans and carrying them out. Both meridians connect to anger, which can show on the face as frowning and narrowed eyes. The related points (Yang Brightness and Pupil Bone) can be used to release resentments of wrongs that we feel have been done to us in the past; in their place appear the seeds of new ideas and thought patterns. As we touch these points, we focus on bringing contentment into our lives, concentrate on feeling balance and harmony, and firmly decide to live a healthy, loving life. During springtime, then, we need to reflect on the new experiences we would like to attract into our lives, especially experiences of inner healing, self-worth, peace, and calm.

The liver is responsible for storing fat and clearing toxic substances from the blood. When we overindulge in food and alcoholic beverages, toxicity can build up in the liver, so give the liver a rest from time to time. Since spring is the season of the liver, it is a great time to do so. Consuming nothing but fresh juice for one day will give the liver the break it needs. Juices such as carrot, beet, and celery are excellent choices for a juice fast, since they help to cleanse the liver. When your liver is happy, your body is happy and you will sleep better, your hormones will be more balanced, and your allergies will be under control.

Symptoms of problems in the gallbladder and liver might include difficulty walking, problems with the eyes, allergies, or hormonal imbalance. A healthy springtime diet to prevent these conditions includes plenty of fresh greens and steamed vegetables, which are high in vitamins and minerals. For a wonderful springtime salad, combine alfalfa sprouts, bean sprouts, avocado, and beet. The antioxidants found in some species of fish help to replenish the cells in the body, so they're a great protein source for the spring. Wild salmon from the Pacific Ocean and Alaska is very high in antioxidants, such as Omega-3 fatty acids.

Springtime Teas

Sassafras tea helps purify the blood, which aids the liver. It's also good for the joints, skin, and kidneys. Dandelion tea is another great springtime healer, since it cleanses the blood and liver. To make either tea, add a small piece of the herb to a stainless steel kettle or pot of water. Soak the herb for 10 to 15 minutes, then bring to a boil, reduce the heat, and simmer for 20 minutes.

Caring for the Eyes

In springtime, we have the opportunity to see things anew; for this reason, spring is the time to concentrate on the eyes. Surprisingly, when we work with the eyes during this season, we not only learn to see our world in a new way, but we can actually improve our eyesight as well! Like springtime, the eyes are linked to the liver and gallbladder meridians.

The Chinese consider the eyes the "window to the soul"; therefore, taking care of them is crucial in Chinese medicine. Your precious eyes truly deserve your loving attention. The eyes are controlled by the liver, so it's important to reduce fat and eliminate alcohol from

Recipe: Congi

Congi (pronounced *con-jee*) is a wonderful dish that combines pork and Chinese yam to both brighten the eyes and strengthen the liver. In the Chinese tradition, Congi fortifies the entire body, while also stimulating the spirit, making it a perfect morning meal. You should be able to find most of the ingredients at a Chinese market.

2 tsp. dried wolfberries (*guo qi zi*) soaked overnight in warm water
2 lb. lean pork (tenderloin), cut into one-inch strips
2 medium pieces dried Chinese yam (*chang yau*)
$3/4$ c. brown or white rice
1 one-inch piece of ginger, peeled and cut in half
2 c. scallions (green onions)
1 tbs. soy sauce
6 c. water

Place water, wolfberries, pork, dried yam, rice, and ginger into a 4-quart enamel soup pot or glass pot. Bring to a boil, then reduce heat and simmer for 25 minutes. Add chopped scallions and soy sauce; return to a boil for about five minutes.

your diet; fat and alcohol can damage the liver, thereby affecting the health of the eyes. When the eyes need refreshing, massage the area just above them and then gently rub the skin next to the inner corners of the eyes. If you are feeling very tired, rub your hands together and then place your palms over your eyes; this will rejuvenate you and give you newfound energy — a new look at life, so to speak.

If you have bags under your eyes, it could be a symptom of congestion in the spleen or kidney. As you improve your digestion by eating warm, nurturing foods and get enough rest, your bags will start to diminish. For puffiness around the eyes, drink water in the morning and afternoon — but not at night — and sleep on a large, fluffy pillow. Investing in the right pillow will ensure you get a good night's sleep, and the result will show in your eyes. You can also reduce puffiness and rest your eyes by making a cup of chrysanthemum or green tea, dipping a cotton ball in the liquid, and placing it on the skin under the eyes. Chrysanthemum tea, whether you drink it or apply it topically as directed above, is also excellent for removing the red from bloodshot eyes.

To stimulate eye rejuvenation, eat wolfberry, known as *guo qi zi* in Chinese; this is available in a dried form in Chinese herbal stores. Also, make sure you have plenty of vitamin A in your diet. Try spending at least ten minutes outdoors every day; the sunlight will stimulate your pituitary gland, benefiting both your brain and eyes. Following is a list of foods for the eyes:

- Fruits: dates, apples, Chinese red or black dates
- Vegetables: aduki beans, dandelion greens, garlic, lotus root (available at Asian food stores), spinach
- Grains: barley, black sesame seeds, brown rice, basmati rice, fennel seeds
- Protein: white fish, such as haddock; tofu
- Herbs: cinnamon, chrysanthemum, wolfberries, ulang tea, garlic, ginger

During spring, take time to relax when you eat. Breathe deeply and chew well. Eat fresh fruits and vegetables, especially green leafy vegetables. Sprout beans while you meditate on what new ideas you want to plant in your life.

Just as farmers monitor the development of their crops as summer approaches, we should pay attention to our own maturation process as we leave springtime in preparation for the busy summer months ahead.

Summer: June 21 to Late August

Summer is the season for growth and maturation. It is also a time for playing, enjoying the outdoors, and rediscovering the child within. Summer is the apex of your energy. It is when you are most active, full of vigor, and able to reach your full potential. Yang energy, the body's most active energy, predominates during this season, so try to embrace it and use it to its maximum capacity for replenishing yourself.

Intuition and creativity play strongly at this time as well. Trusting your intuition allows your heart to be nourished and open to self-love.

The meridians of summer are the heart, small intestine, heart protector, and Triple Warmer:

- The heart is considered the supreme ruler in Chinese medicine; it oversees the entire body.

- The small intestine separates ideas from decisions and helps to cast away clutter and old ideas. The small intestine aids in digestion, of both food and thoughts; biologically it helps filter food, and spiritually it filters negative thoughts. The small intestine meridian ends on the face in front of the ear in the hollow of the cheekbone, and as you touch this point, you can influence your digestive tract. If your small intestine is blocked or not moving properly, you will receive little nourishment from the food you eat; symptoms might include gas and belching. Repeating negative thoughts in your head can be another indication that your small intestine is blocked.

- The heart protector is the pericardium, a membrane that surrounds the heart; it not only protects the heart but also helps to resolve old conflicts of self-doubt.

- The Triple Warmer is connected to your endocrine system and helps your immune system stay healthy. It starts on the outside of the fourth finger, goes up the outside of the arm and ends by the outer corner of the eyebrow.

According to traditional Chinese medicine, joy is the emotion of summer and its meridians. Joy can be found in simple things such as listening to music or simply being quiet and reflecting on life. Or it can be found in more yang activities, such as playing sports, practicing yoga, or dancing. Most especially, joy found in nature connects to the inner spirit. In summertime, take walks in nature, for this brings joy and stimulates the heart.

The diet of summer includes fresh fruits in the morning and vegetables later in the day. Start the day with hot water and lemon, which cleanses the liver and nourishes the heart. Since it is the hottest season, eat plenty of cooling foods: lots of fruit, especially berries, which are high in antioxidants; vegetables, such as fresh salads at room temperature and warm mustard greens; whole grains such as rice, buckwheat, and millet; seeds and nuts; and a small amount of lean meat, poultry, or fish.

Summertime Teas

Peppermint and comfrey teas are excellent cooling teas for this hot time of year. They are available at natural food stores.

Hawthorn berry tea strengthens the heart. Add 2 ounces of hawthorn berries to 1 quart of boiling water, reduce heat, and steep for 10 minutes. Drink a cup of this tea once or twice a day.

Spices like cayenne pepper and ginger strengthen the heart. Cauliflower, cabbage, and garlic stimulate the heart as well. To feed the small intestine, combine one cup each of sunflower seeds, lentils, and brown rice in a large pot. Add six cups of water, bring to a boil, reduce heat, and simmer for forty-five minutes. Licorice root and fennel seed stimulate the small intestine as well.

In the summer it is especially important to minimize your intake of dairy products, fried foods, and processed foods since they're so heavy and difficult to digest. Also, try not to mix different kinds of foods, for this produces gas, which is hard on the digestive tract.

As summer comes to a close, you can feel your energy wane as you approach Indian Summer.

Indian Summer: Final Days of August to September 21

During Indian summer you prepare for autumn. It is the beginning of harvest time, the season of the earth, a time when we receive support and nutrients and ready ourselves to rest and reflect. It is a time for being grounded, for gathering the seeds of richness. Indian summer is a transitional time, a time for shedding stress and becoming centered, a season for evaluating life and connecting with the core essence.

Indian summer is the season of the stomach and spleen, organs that rule over the earth. The earth gives us the power to form thoughts and to manifest our intentions, and it relates to the intake of nourishment. The stomach and spleen relate to nurturing the self through nature and to playing with friends. These meridians are partners; the primary stomach meridian starts on the face under the eye, and it feeds the spleen meridian. The stomach meridian has forty-four points along its pathway and influences digestion on a mental and physical level. The spleen is vital to proper digestion, since it links all the organs together and supports the transportation of nutrients to every part of the body. By nurturing the spleen, you are regulating the intestinal tract.

The emotion the stomach and spleen meridians share is worry or overthinking. Obsessiveness and the despair brought on by dwelling on problems are the emotional conditions present when there is an imbalance between stomach and spleen. These conditions show in the face as worry lines, tightness and tension, and general stress. The lips can indicate stomach and spleen imbalance as well; they peel and crack and appear to have lines around them. A yellow tinge on the sides of the face can also indicate a problem with the spleen.

Indian Summer Teas

Chamomile tea is great at this time of year, for it stimulates the stomach and calms the nervous system. Other herbs that are good for the stomach include thyme, ginseng, and clove, while parsley, dandelion, and chicory bolster the spleen.

Cardamom and fennel tea is also helpful during Indian summer because it aids digestion. Steep for 15 minutes and let sit for 15 minutes before drinking. Or try peppermint tea, an old standby for healthy digestion.

Foods such as millet, mallow, and beef or ox are all good for the stomach and spleen. Proper nourishment might also include fruit in the morning, followed a half-hour later with protein or a cereal. Yellow and orange foods such as summer squash and pumpkin, as well as seeds, fish, and poultry, are also appropriate for this season.

As you leave Indian summer you begin to go inside yourself as you approach autumn.

Autumn: September 21 to December 20

September 21 marks a day to reflect on the blessings of summer and to begin preparing for winter. Autumn is the season of harvest, the fruition of your inner and outer growth. Everything you have sown you will now reap. It is a time to complete projects, to shed unwanted thoughts of negativity, to replenish the soul, and to reclaim personal power. This is a time for prayer and meditation and for listening closely to your inner guidance, your intuition. It is a time to relax, a season for spending quiet time in nature and for healing. In autumn, we begin to turn inward and redirect our energy toward reflection and gratitude for who and what are important to us.

Autumn controls the pathways of the lungs and the colon (large intestine). These organs are stimulated by applying gentle pressure to a point next to the nose. The lungs have to do with new ideas and thoughts, and healthy lungs also mean beautiful skin. The lungs, not surprisingly, are associated with breathing — more specifically, breathing with our connectedness to the God-self. As you inhale, you breathe in spiritual or heavenly essence. Diaphragmatic, or "belly," breathing opens your core to your spiritual essence. As you become better able to observe the breath, you become a keen observer of your own thoughts. This is a meditative process based in contemplative reflection. Many use the process of breathing — in through the nose and out through the mouth — in the early morning for centering the self and preparing for the day.

The colon meridian starts on the outside of the index finger, goes along the outer edge of the arm, and ends on the face, next to the nose. The colon has to do with elimination, on the physical, mental, and spiritual levels. On the physical level its job is to let go of waste, while on the mental and spiritual levels it facilitates letting go of the past. This meridian is also linked to the energy of "father," whether earthly or heavenly, and marks a time in which to resolve issues with the father and bring harmony to the family within.

The emotion of autumn and its meridians is grief, so if there is a death or mourning process in progress, you should focus on the lung and colon pathways, concentrating on letting go of grief, especially the sorrows connected with the past. Unexpressed emotions such as anger or depression can block the colon, so try to communicate these feelings and then let them go.

The Chinese book of wisdom, the Nei Ching, says that the large intestine is like the official who propagates the right way of living. Autumn, then, is a good time for body cleansing, which might include loofah skin brushing, colon hydrotherapy, and shifting the diet.

Consuming warm foods, such as squash and pumpkin, is ideal in autumn, while dairy products and processed foods, which can block the colon, are to be avoided. Also, be careful not to eat too much meat in the fall, since an excess of meat can stress the colon. Eat less fruit now as the weather gets colder; however, apples are great in the fall since they are in season and they cleanse the colon. This is a great time for squash soup or other vegetable soups, lightly steamed vegetables, and whole grains, all of which will assist with healthy elimination and keep the intestines well toned. Pungent curries may be too harsh in this season.

Autumn Teas

Burdock root tea is great in the autumn, for it works as a tonic for the colon. Cascara sagrada tea works as a laxative, cleansing the colon.

Coltsfoot and mullen teas act as a lung tonic. Other teas for the lungs include slippery elm, horehound, and yerba sante.

Licorice root makes an excellent autumn tea, for it stimulates both the colon and the lungs.

Grapes are healthy in autumn, for they can act as a tonic for the lungs and colon. Garlic is another healthy autumn food, for it aids in cleansing the lungs. Spruce up your autumn salads by adding one tablespoon of cold-pressed olive oil, which promotes healthy intestinal function, and one tablespoon of ground flax seed, which will aid digestion.

It is important to stay dry during fall to protect the lungs, and to have a bowel movement each day in order to eliminate toxins.

As you leave autumn, you will experience your energy going deep inside yourself.

Winter: December 21 to March 20

Winter is the season for nesting, for going deep within, for hibernating. It is the critical time of year for the deep rest that brings replenishment. It is also a season for looking ahead to see clearly what you want to bring into your life. It is important to stay warm and dry during winter.

As you dream during this season, you get in touch with old family traditions. In focusing on your ancestral lineage, you renew your spirit. Listen for messages of love, appreciation, and healing that you may be whispering to yourself. In winter you are most receptive to new thoughts, and your willpower fortifies the soul to get done what needs doing.

Winter is the season of the kidney and bladder meridians, which are connected to the bones and replenished by the element of water. The human body is about 65 percent water. Water helps to circulate the blood and lymphatic fluids and also helps to eliminate waste. The kidneys store life energy and are related to inner and outer transformation. They also control the ears and hearing, the bones and bone marrow, the teeth, spine, and knees. Also, the kidneys and bladder are connected to birth, conception, and the reproductive system. Because they have to do with birthing new ideas and possessing the willpower to follow through, the kidneys control your brain and your thoughts. The kidneys' partner, the bladder meridian, begins in the inner canthus, or corner of the eye, and goes over the top of the head and then alongside the spine. It goes through every organ in the body and ends on the outside of the little toe. There are sixty-seven points along this pathway. The bladder meridian influences fluid retention.

Fear is the emotion of the kidneys and bladder, and this fear can manifest as a phobia or anxiety. You can learn to let go of fear through love. Long-term illnesses, lower-back stiffness, and blue-black circles under the eyes can be related to kidney imbalance. Conversely, when your eyes sparkle, the life force related to your kidneys is strong. Longevity is also controlled by the kidneys.

The diet during the winter should be rich in warm, nurturing foods. Vegetable soups and root vegetables such as turnips, garlic, and ginger should be used during the winter. Cooked grains of millet, brown rice, or adzuki beans are good for the kidneys. Deep-sea fish like sea bass are excellent sources of protein. Seaweed is also good during the winter, since it contains large quantities of the minerals needed to stimulate the endocrine system. Beware of too much salt, which can injure the kidneys and raise blood pressure.

As winter comes to a close, the seeds that have lain dormant start to come alive in preparation for the vibrance of spring. Similarly, you will begin to rub the sleep from your eyes and emerge from your hibernation.

Wintertime Teas

Marshmallow root promotes health in the kidneys and bladder and acts as a diuretic. To make it, steep the root for 15 to 20 minutes. Nettle tea also acts as a diuretic and is good for the kidneys. Fenugreek is another, and it functions also as an adrenal tonic.

Juniper berries help to strengthen the kidneys. Combine them in a tea with uvi ursi, an herb that stimulates the bladder.

IT IS MY HOPE THAT AS YOU UNDERSTAND the importance of the seasons and begin to live according to them, your life will settle into its own natural rhythms. Things go smoothly when you learn to not push against the flow of nature.

In the next chapter we will discuss another of Mother Nature's gifts, the magic of essential oils — one more component of your healthy new lifestyle.

CHAPTER EIGHT

The Magic of Essential Oils

Essential oils — subtle, highly concentrated plant oils distilled from shrubs, flowers, and trees — have been a natural and necessary part of beauty routines worldwide for millennia. In ancient Egypt, such oils were used to keep the skin healthy and youthful and to stimulate inspiration. In the Bible, Psalm 133 refers to both myrrh and frankincense, essential oils that were used to anoint the faithful. Today the use of essential oils for self-care is known as aromatherapy.

Essential oils are absorbed into the body either through the skin or by inhalation. They work on many different levels: physical, psychological, emotional, and spiritual. Since they stimulate the sense of smell and are absorbed through the skin, they can reach any part of the body within minutes.

On the physical level, essential oils can transform the entire body into an instrument of health. They can oxygenate the cells and help transport nutrients throughout the body. Also, they can help improve digestion and open the sinuses. By increasing circulation, hydration, and waste removal, many essential oils help the body rejuvenate and regenerate at the cellular level. They can regulate, invigorate, and stabilize the function of internal organs, and they stimulate the lymphatic system, which clarifies the skin and helps to bring out one's inner beauty.

On the emotional level, essential oils can enhance well-being and aid in the process of release. Some oils can be used to stimulate moods, while others work wonders for relaxation. Lavender, for example, is a wonderfully relaxing oil. Sometimes I use it in my facial masks or have clients inhale it, for it goes directly to the olfactory area of the brain and helps to relax them. As you smell the oils, your body will open to greater relaxation and healing.

Many of the oils are too strong to be used alone, so you must dilute them in a base oil before applying them to your skin. Sweet almond oil is a great oil for this purpose. When applied to the skin, essential oils can help diminish wrinkles and restore elasticity. Also, they can help reduce stress lines and puffiness and keep collagen in good condition. You can add essential oils to the Acupressure Facelift routine by dabbing the diluted oils onto the acupressure points or by using a diffuser (available at herbal and natural food stores), which uses the heat of a candle flame to vaporize the oil. The aromas of the oils can both increase the effectiveness of the Facelift and make the Facelift more enjoyable for you. There are numerous oils to choose from for your facial rejuvenation program. Below you'll find a list of oils and their properties.

Many brands of essential oils are available in natural food and holistic health care stores, as well as online. In my practice I use oils manufactured by Young Living, for I find them to be some of the purest oils available.

A List of Essential Oils and Their Benefits

Angelica root

Body: Fights fatigue, stress, and headaches; aids digestion and illness recovery; cleanses blood.

Mind: Relaxes nerves; creates stability; releases negative feelings.

Spirit: Provides protection and courage; harmonizes body, mind, and spirit; rebuilds the soul.

Basil

Body: Reduces fever; eases congestion; releases muscle spasm; helps migraines.

Mind: Boosts confidence and courage; clears the mind; stimulates the brain; increases memory.

Spirit: Protects the soul.

Bergamot

Body: Relieves PMS, menopause symptoms, candida, and urinary and respiratory infections.
Mind: Relieves fear and anger; reduces mood swings and depression.
Spirit: Opens the heart essence to love and light; radiates joy and healing to others.

Black pepper

Body: Heals bruising; stimulates appetite; strengthens entire system.
Mind: Relieves anger; boosts mental activity; stimulates alertness and memory.
Spirit: Grounds spirit into the physical; balances spirit and emotions.

Cedarwood

Body: Acts as general tonic, antiseptic, astringent, diuretic, expectorant.
Mind: Strengthens and fortifies will and wisdom; calms tension.
Spirit: Promotes grounding and clarity; dispels negative energy; connects to the divine.

Cinnamon bark

Body: Calms muscle spasms and painful joints; relieves cold and flu symptoms.
Mind: Treats exhaustion and depression; acts as an aphrodisiac.
Spirit: Warms and arouses the spirit.

Clary sage

Body: Eases PMS and menopausal disorders; relieves asthma.
Mind: Relieves anxiety and emotional tension; promotes deep sleep.
Spirit: Activates centering, grounding, balancing, recharging,
  awakening, inspiration.

Clove

Body: Prevents contagious illnesses; eases toothaches; stimulates
  digestion.
Mind: Lifts depression; dispels lethargy; relieves anxiety; stimulates
  memory.
Spirit: Protects the spirit and promotes universal love and beauty.

Cypress

Body: Acts as antiseptic, antispasmodic, astringent, deodorant,
  diuretic, decongestant; aids the lymphatic system.
Mind: Provides stability; facilitates letting go and coping with
  change and grief.
Spirit: Promotes transformation.

Eucalyptus

Body: Supports respiratory system; strengthens immune system;
  helps with herpes.
Mind: Reduces mood swings.
Spirit: Stimulates a wider perception of life.

Fennel

Body: Enhances hearing and eyesight; stimulates circulatory and respiratory systems.
Mind: Relaxes the mind; promotes strength, courage, and creativity.
Spirit: Promotes confidence and self-expression.

Frankincense

Body: Acts as antitumoral and expectorant; stimulates immune system; eliminates ringworm.
Mind: Relieves depression; calms the mind and emotions.
Spirit: Provides spiritual self-discipline; expands consciousness.

Geranium

Body: Soothes dry skin; regulates menstrual cycle and hormones; relieves PMS.
Mind: Eases anxiety, depression, mood swings, frustration, and irritability.
Spirit: Lifts the spirit; encourages imagination, intuition, and sensory experience.

Ginger

Body: Aids appetite and digestion; treats nausea, travel sickness, colds, and sore throats.
Mind: Sharpens the senses; activates willpower; stimulates initiative; restores determination.
Spirit: Grounds the spirit, connecting it to the physical body.

Grapefruit

Body: Detoxifies; aids blood circulation; treats oily skin and acne.
Mind: Eases depression and moodiness; relieves frustration.
Spirit: Promotes lightness of spirit.

Helichrysum (aka Everlasting)

Body: Aids digestion; relieves migraines, skin problems; reduces
scarring; acts as anticoagulant.
Mind: Stimulates dream activity; elevates mood; alleviates tension
and frustration.
Spirit: Activates intuition; dissolves negativity; promotes compassion.

Hyssop

Body: Works as a disinfectant; stimulates lungs; restores vitality.
Mind: Invigorates the mind; improves concentration; relieves pessimism.
Spirit: Promotes spiritual insight.

Jasmine

Body: Eases frigidity, impotence, and nervous anxiety.
Mind: Instills confidence, optimism, energy, and emotional balance.
Spirit: Restores values on the soul level.

Juniper

Body: Helps rheumatic pain; soothes and hydrates dry skin;
stimulates kidneys.

Mind: Relieves worry; overcomes depression; promotes self-esteem.
Spirit: Purifies the spirit.

Lavender

Body: Treats burns, dermatitis, eczema, psoriasis, boils, and acne; restores the skin's elasticity.
Mind: Soothes anxiety and fear; eases anger, frustration, and headaches.
Spirit: Promotes renewal and inspiration.

Lemon

Body: Stops bleeding; treats gums, gingivitis, and mouth ulcers.
Mind: Helps ability to memorize; brings in optimism and humor.
Spirit: Opens heart center; uplifts spirit.

Lemongrass

Body: Soothes headaches; repels insects; lowers fever; protects against staph infections.
Mind: Relieves stress; lifts the spirit.
Spirit: Enhances psychic awareness.

Marjoram

Body: Removes muscle and joint pain; helps with asthma, bronchitis, and sinusitis.

Mind: Calms obsessive thinking and neediness; helps one to
   accept loss.
Spirit: Clears psychic pathways.

Melissa/Lemon Balm

Body: Calms upset stomachs; calms heart; lowers blood pressure;
   manages herpes.
Mind: Calms hysteria, shock, and panic; removes mental blocks.
Spirit: Soothes inner child.

Myrhh

Body: Regenerates skin; stimulates thyroid; regulates hormones; acts
   as antioxidant and anti-inflammatory.
Mind: Clears the mind; stimulates the memory and emotions.
Spirit: Puts you in touch with your spiritual essence, your God-self;
   promotes spiritual awareness.

Myrtle

Body: For use with urinary infections, acne, hemorrhoids, children's
   cough.
Mind: Relieves addictions and self-destructive behaviors.
Spirit: Opens access to stored knowledge; aligns energy centers.

Neroli

Body: Helps insomnia; stimulates digestive system; strengthens veins.

Mind: Eases depression and anxiety; stabilizes and releases emotions.

Spirit: Connects body and mind; balances male and female with heart energies.

Nutmeg

Body: Treats digestive and kidney problems; awakens new strength and vitality.

Mind: Encourages flexibility and detachment; eases pain of loss.

Spirit: Provides liberation and comfort.

Orange

Body: Eases indigestion, nausea, vomiting, constipation, and irritable bowel; stimulates liver.

Mind: Promotes mental clarity and emotional balance.

Spirit: Transforms and repairs energy centers and the auric field.

Oregano

Body: In a poultice, treats scorpion and spider bites; helps toothaches and many skin problems.

Mind: Mental tonic; calms and cleanses.

Spirit: Protects the energy field.

Patchouli

Body: Stimulates regrowth of skin cells; heals rough, cracked skin and wounds.

Mind: Alleviates the blues; quiets an overactive intellect.

Spirit: Aligns root, sacral, and heart energy centers.

Peppermint

Body: Relieves fevers, colds, flu, motion sickness, headaches, nausea, and digestive disorders.

Mind: Invigorates mind and concentration; stimulates mental alertness and focus.

Spirit: Refreshes the spirit; inspires discernment.

Pine

Body: Reduces gall stones; helps poor circulation and kidney and bladder problems.

Mind: Helps with nervous exhaustion; restores emotional boundaries.

Spirit: Protects and clears energy centers.

Rose

Body: Strengthens the heart, circulation, and digestion; regenerates skin.

Mind: Helps with postnatal depression, sadness and grief, and relationship issues.

Spirit: Expands the heart and crown energy centers to allow unconditional love.

Rosemary

Body: Lowers cholesterol levels in blood; helps with muscle stiffness and cramping.

Mind: Enhances concentration and mental clarity; restores self-worth.

Spirit: Strengthens spiritual path and values; assists with recalling past lives; provides protection.

Rosewood

Body: Acts as antidepressant, antiseptic, bactericide, improves the skin's elasticity.

Mind: Relieves anxiety, depression, and moodiness.

Spirit: Provides patience for divine timing; dissolves energy blocks.

Sandalwood

Body: Relieves dehydrated, itchy, and inflamed skin; acts as astringent for oily skin.

Mind: Reduces tension, confusion, fear, and stress.

Spirit: Enhances meditation and spiritual practices; aligns body, mind, and spirit.

Tarragon

Body: Overcomes shock; expels worms and mucous; acts as liver cleanser.

Mind: Clears confusion and stabilizes emotions; shines light on dark issues.

Spirit: Repairs aura; removes old energy patterns.

Tea tree

Body: Treats skin infections, burns, wounds, athlete's foot, warts, and other skin problems; relieves candida; good for teeth and gum disease; eases water retention and hypertension.

Mind: Enhances confidence and mental strength; relieves mental fatigue and depression.

Spirit: Cleans and heals openings in energy centers.

Thyme

Body: Relieves pain from arthritis; stimulates digestion, kidneys, lungs, and nervous system.

Mind: Dispels melancholy; stimulates strength and confidence; invigorates memory.

Spirit: Stimulates senses of courage, security, love, and compassion.

Vetiver

Body: Eases joint pain and inflammatory problems; helps with eating disorders; balances hormones.

Mind: Relaxes and soothes emotions and overactive minds.
Spirit: Brings together spiritual and physical energies.

Ylang ylang

Body: Treats skin conditions, eating disorders, and high blood pressure; stimulates hair growth; regulates heartbeat; acts as antiparasitic.
Mind: Dispels fear of intimacy; eases depression, insomnia, anxiety, and low self-esteem; combats anger; improves mental focus.
Spirit: Balances male and female energies; restores confidence and peace.

Essential Oil Skin-Care Recipes

Here are a couple of recipes for essential oil blends to treat your skin.

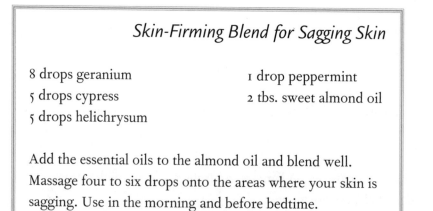

Skin-Firming Blend for Sagging Skin

8 drops geranium
5 drops cypress
5 drops helichrysum

1 drop peppermint
2 tbs. sweet almond oil

Add the essential oils to the almond oil and blend well. Massage four to six drops onto the areas where your skin is sagging. Use in the morning and before bedtime.

Anti-Wrinkle Treatment

5 drops sandalwood   5 drops lavender

5 drops helichrysum   5 drops frankincense

5 drops geranium   2 tbs. sweet almond oil

Add essential oils to almond oil and blend well. Apply to wrinkle-prone areas. Be careful not to get the product in your eyes.

ONCE YOU START EXPERIMENTING with essential oils, you'll be amazed at how they help you look and feel better. In the next chapter, we'll explore several more tools to enhance your well-being.

CHAPTER NINE

Your Healthy New Lifestyle

In these pages, we've covered a lot of ground, and by now you've probably realized that the Acupressure Facelift is just one facet of a healthy, balanced lifestyle. When you adopt the practices covered in this book — holistic skin care, acupressure, proper nutrition, seasonal living, the use of essential oils, and those we'll cover in this chapter — your divine essence will emerge to reveal a bright, shining you.

Now let's look at some more pieces of the puzzle, including journaling, proper rest, healthy sexual habits, physical exercise, qigong and tai chi chih, self-massage, the Hawaiian spirit of Aloha, the power of positive thinking, and focusing your life. The information I offer on these subjects is basic and meant solely to introduce you to them; to learn more, I recommend you do some research on the Internet or search for books at your local library or favorite personal-care bookstore.

Journaling

Writing in a journal is a wonderful way to process your life experiences, work through negative or painful emotions, and remind yourself of the many things you have to be grateful for. When you write in a journal, you are taking time to stop and reflect in order to grow. Journaling is a wonderful way to release negative memories and to help focus on new joy, peacefulness, and healing in your life. Try to make a regular practice of journaling, sitting down to write every morning or evening for five, ten, twenty minutes — whatever you can manage. You'll be amazed at how this process facilitates personal growth and connects you to your divine spirit.

Experiment with journaling as part of your Acupressure Facelift routine. When you touch a specific point, notice how it makes you feel, and then write about it. Use the suggested affirmations for each point as a springboard for your writing.

Rest

It is important to stop and rest before you become exhausted. Taking frequent short breaks during the day is critical to conserving energy. At night, you should go to sleep on an empty stomach before ten o'clock. Retiring after ten can cause the energy of the liver to rise, which can produce a "second wind" that makes it more difficult to get to sleep.

Turn off the TV well before bedtime, and refrain from reading the news of the day before going to sleep; what you see and what you read will affect the dream state, and most of the news is negative. Your dream state is the time during which you contact the spirit world and set the tone for creating your life scene, so you want to enter it with as little baggage from the day as possible.

To counter any negative energies that could disrupt your sleep, relax before bedtime by writing a gratitude list, writing in your journal, or perhaps drinking chamomile tea. When retiring, it is important to reflect on what has been positive that day, then calm your mind and relax your eyes.

Moderation in Sex

Having just enough sex — neither too much nor too little — is a key to vitality. Too much sex can injure your *jing*, or ancestral energy. It can also harm the kidneys. Pacing your sexual activity is essential.

Spring is the time of year when sexual activity reaches its apex. During summer sexual activity begins to decline, and it continues to do so throughout autumn. In winter, the time of quiescence, there is further tapering off. Winter is also the time for the kidneys to recuperate and prepare for the new energy that spring will bring, and this parallel between sexual energy and the activity of the kidneys demonstrates the natural connection between the two.

Exercise

Physical exercise in an integral part of a healthy lifestyle. Lack of exercise causes disease, for it impairs circulation of chi and blood, weakens the stomach, and saps energy. When you sit for too long, your system tends to become sluggish — and this is true for both body and mind. Regular exercise, on the other hand, boosts energy and does wonders for overall health.

Regularity and persistence are important in exercise. You should get some exercise every day. If you're not accustomed to strenuous activity, start out by taking a walk every day. Twenty minutes is sufficient to get the chi moving, but you can increase this duration as your schedule and fitness level permit.

Aerobic exercise, such as walking, running, cycling, swimming, and many team sports, strengthens the heart. Lifting weights and doing abdominal crunches help to keep muscles taut and trim and boost the metabolism. Stretching keeps the joints open and helps the flow of blood. Relaxing with each breath and breathing into all parts of the body keeps all parts flowing smoothly and evenly.

Qigong and Tai Chi Chih

In addition to the forms of exercise mentioned above, you may improve your energy through qigong, an ancient Chinese system of exercises that stimulate the flow of chi, or vital energy, along the meridians. The qigong tradition emphasizes the importance of remaining well. It cultivates inner strength, calms the mind, and restores the body to its natural state of health by maintaining optimum functioning of all body systems.

The practice of qigong can be used to preserve health and regenerate the spirit. Qigong is based on breathing, movement, and visualization, and it can be performed both sitting and standing. Through qigong, you can manufacture and circulate chi more effectively in order to bathe those areas that need healing. Qigong emphasizes deep breathing to calm the mind, relieve stress, and massage the internal organs.

You can further replenish yourself and help promote longevity through the ancient Chinese program of exercises called tai chi chih, a form of qigong. The gentle exercises — which can be performed by almost anyone, regardless of physical fitness — combine mental concentration, coordinated breathing, and slow, graceful body movements to increase well-being, lessen stress, and strengthen the body. Tai chi chih stimulates and balances the flow of chi. It cultivates inner strength, calms the mind, and restores the body to a natural state of health by maintaining optimum functioning of all body systems.

If possible, do tai chi once a day, preferably in the morning. However, it is best to not practice while you are menstruating. You should eat about two hours prior to your practice (that is, do not practice on a full stomach), and your meal should consist of nourishment that provides the best fuel, notably fruits and vegetables. While practicing, you should wear comfortable clothing and remove all adornments such as jewelry.

Qigong and tai chi are stimulators, so do not practice them before bedtime. And if possible, practice in fresh outdoor air. Keep the spirit calm and peaceful while engaging in these exercises.

Self-Massage

Self-massage promotes the flow of energy within your body that keeps you vibrant and healthy. Here are some simple techniques:

- Move your lower jaw back and forth. This allows for the flow of energy from the yin to the yang, and the resulting vibration activates the brain.

- Massage your hands and scalp to stimulate all parts of the body, revitalizing the internal organs and bodily functions.

- Massage your ears to activate the internal organs.

- Gently massage the area just below your navel, called the Sea of Energy, or *Don Tien*, to rekindle your internal fire. (This area of the body is also called the Lower Burner.)

- Rub the base of your spine, or sacrum, eighteen times to bring warmth to the adrenals and activate the kidneys; stimulating the kidneys is the key to longevity in Chinese medicine. Rubbing your lower back also helps you stay balanced in the nervous system and helps with your metabolism.

- Massage your belly in a clockwise direction while lying on your right side; this will aid digestion and stimulate the colon to promote healthy bowel movements. It will also help diminish the facial lines going from your nose to your mouth.

- Rub your midback to stimulate the *mingmen*, or Gate of Life. This will keep the kidneys vital.

- Massage your skull to enliven the brain. The point at the top of the head is called *Bai Wei*, or Point of Thousand-Petaled Lotus. Massaging this point connects you to the heavenly energy and brings you closer to nirvana, or enlightenment. Massage this point nine times in a circular motion.

- Rub the bottoms of your feet to ground yourself in earthly energy. As you do this, you strengthen the entire body.

- Massage your joints; this will keep you limber, since wherever you have a joint, the chi and blood can get stuck.

The Power of Visualization

Using visualization techniques while you exercise, practice qigong or tai chi, or perform self-massage can help to recharge and regenerate the body. If you visualize the energy coming up the Governor Vessel (the spine) and down the Conception Vessel (front), all of your meridians will be regenerated and your yin and yang energies will be balanced.

The Spirit of Aloha

Chinese medicine entered our Western culture by way of Hawaii, which has served as the gateway for Eastern cultures to enter the West. When the Chinese brought their philosophy to the islands and began to study the ancient Hawaiian traditions and culture, they found many avenues for cultural integration.

The Hawaiian Aloha spirit is a way of life in which one lives from the heart. Practitioners of Aloha principles learn to let go of fear and realign themselves with their spiritual essence. As the soul comes forth, the practitioner learns to tune in to his or her birthright, which is an innate trust of instincts and a conscious development of the powers of intuition. Reconnecting with nature is also an important element of Hawaiian spirituality.

The Hawaiian spiritual tradition returns us to simplicity and a sharing of life, with the realization that we are all one. As we live with this awareness we replenish ourselves at a cellular level; we let go of past conditioning and bring peace and balance into our lives and into the world around us. We connect to the God within, and when we do, each and every cell vibrates in harmony. Learning to trust the self and live from love allows the body to function at an optimal level. The face shines, the eyes glow, and we come to live with an internal smile that shows on our face, decreasing lines and exuding radiance.

I have had the opportunity to spend time with two great Hawaiian teachers, or *Kahunas*, as they are called — Papa Kei and Auntie Poepoe. Both were simple people who saw the oneness in everything.

The message from both was the same: trust your intuition, live with compassion, and live from your heart.

This Aloha Spirit permeated everything they did, and they gave love, compassion, and joy to the community. They practiced Hawaiian massage and knew everything about Hawaiian plants, because they knew that being connected to the environment is a key to wellness. They never said no to anyone who crossed their paths.

The Power of Positive Thinking

How you organize your thoughts and keep a clear mind has much to do with mental and spiritual regeneration. Every thought and word consumes energy. When one overthinks or worries, then fatigue — even exhaustion and overall ill health — will result. Clear your mind of negative thoughts. Think instead of the positive.

Every thought we have sends an electrical charge to the rest of the body, a message that will either deplete us or nourish us, depending on whether that message is negative or positive. When negative thoughts produce ill feelings, the body stops working properly, and consequently digestion gets disrupted; bones become thin and brittle; the skin ages and shrivels, because it isn't producing elastin.

Not only do our thoughts affect our own physicality, but they also radiate to others in our circle of family and friends and beyond. This phenomenon matters very much, because through our thoughts, we are creating the quality of our lives and the lives of those around us.

This phenomenon occurs because we are all connected to each other. We really are all one, and nothing happens outside of us that does not affect us on the inside, at any place or in any time. Conversely, what happens inside also shows up on the outside.

What do you want your thoughts to be like? And what on earth can you do about negative thoughts and ideas?

The most profound belief you could ever have is that you can choose your very thoughts. Just as our bodies are made up of large amounts of water that are mutable, so, too, our thoughts are changeable. A negative thought can easily be transformed into a positive one, so that new, greater experiences evolve, and our lives transform into the "love lives" we were meant to have.

When you hear your own negative messages, you can say to yourself, "Stop...clear." This is an easy way to interrupt negative energy. Every time you interrupt a thought you don't want to have, you change your perspective and shift your world toward positivity and love.

There are many ways to turn negatives into positives: listening to soothing music; exchanging ideas and conversation with like-minded, positive people; taking quiet time to love and appreciate yourself; finding patience for yourself; expressing gratitude; and reading positive material — all these behaviors will help to create a loving and nurturing space in your life. As you learn to dream and gain knowledge that inspires you, you will help stop negative patterns from enveloping you.

The only way you can ever be great is to take control of your mind. As you create your life each day in beauty, you transform the planet into a garden of peace, love, and calm. You are here to infiltrate the cosmos with your ideas. Your purpose is to develop your gifts of intentionality to transform your life and live your greatness. When you do, your face will glow with your inner beingness; your eyes will sparkle and radiate self-love.

Finding Focus in Your Life

Create positive ideals. Establish your own values and let go of a life of complacency. When you lead a mundane life, in which all your activities are routine and uninspiring, your soul never has the opportunity to rise to the surface. But when you ask yourself instead, "What is my purpose?" and "Is there something more?" your soul lights up, for you are surrounding yourself with a newness.

When you focus on worldly problems, you become dull and lifeless, and you send a death-thought to every cell. But as you realign with spirit, your cells are replenished, reprogrammed with new thoughts. Every cell becomes electrically alive as you feed to your nerve endings new messages that are then transported to every cell. This, then, is the way to rewire your brain and change your thoughts. Only you can make the choices to break habits of boredom and frustration, to strive for the new and to dream a life of self-worth that imparts an inner beauty for all to see.

As you focus on a particular desire in your life, you help to bring all the invisible forces in the universe into focus on a single concrete point. When you are inspired to take care of and rejuvenate yourself, all the forces in your body gather to support this concentration of belief. As you take time to breathe, meditate, and focus on spiritual, mental, and physical renewal, your cells hear these thoughts and register them in your brain, which sends a powerful message to your nerve endings. Your body responds accordingly.

Take time out of each day — or better yet, each hour — to reconnect with your higher, spiritual self and focus on your intentions of self-improvement and wholeness. Doing so will turn these intentions into reality. As your inner reaches are bathed in these new thoughts, you will find rest, calm, and inner nourishment, and you will become less attached to the outer world. You will become your own source, and you will no longer need to play victim to life's circumstances. You will become renewed, rejuvenated, and replenished, for your soul is in control.

Some Final Thoughts

1. Take time daily to reconnect with spirit.

2. Trust your inner knowing and intuition. You will become balanced and will move forward with a sense of trust and well-being.

3. Love yourself and love spirit. Realize that we are all one. This awareness is critical to inner rejuvenation and self-mastery.

4. Surrender to spirit and trust your inner guidance. This magnificent commitment is a step to cellular rejuvenation and renewal.

5. Pray. Prayer is a concrete way to know that all is possible.

6. Practice affirmations: I am the face of God and become replenished as I connect to my God-self.

7. Appreciate yourself and all who come into your life. Write a gratitude list daily.

8. Be willing in all things. Willingness is the key to awakening your potential.

9. Let go of doubt and fear; all parts of your inner being will then realign with wellness and appreciation for who and what you are.

10. Look at the perfection of a flower and see in it your own perfection.

11. Imagine. Imagination is the link to focusing your thoughts.

12. Radiate peace. As you become peaceful, your soul aligns with spirit, producing health, harmony, and peace of mind.

THIS IS THE BEGINNING OF YOUR NEW LIFE. As you absorb the information in this book, stop, listen, and feel yourself beginning to be transformed. Now apply your new process of gentleness and calm to all aspects of your life. Walk forward with dignity and grace, and realize that you are a special, angelic child of God. Treat yourself gently, and regard each person you meet with love and kindness. As you transform yourself, you will truly transform the world.

Acknowledgments

Thanks to Mary Betts for her support and encouragement; to David Nanney for the interior photos; to Fay Marley-Clarke for her photography and design; to Lea Schoenwetter for her design and editing; to Theresa Barbera-Aiken for her countless contributions far and wide; and to Michaela Safadi and Diane Cummings for their editing.

Very special acknowledgments go to Mary Elizabeth Wakefield and Sunanda Stokes for waking me up to the gifts of facial acupressure; to Spa Luna in Maui, Hawaii, for my training in skin care; to RainStar University of Complementary and Alternative Medicine, where I will be teaching facial rejuvenation training programs; to the dear and wonderful Jo Ann De Lora; to Katar for being who she is; to Marcella Vonn Harting; and finally, to Angela Mattey for her unrelenting support and caring.

My deepest gratitude goes to the team at New World Library. Collaborating with such a professional and visionary company on this labor of love has been a joy. Thanks to Georgia Hughes for our connection and her patience and friendship; to Kristen Cashman for her tireless editing and attention to detail; to Kim Corbin for enthusiastically publicizing the book; to Tona Pearce Myers for the graceful interior design and typesetting; and to Tracy Pitts for the gorgeous cover.

About the Author

Victoria Mogilner, C.A., is a Chinese medicine practitioner and a certified acupuncturist, aesthetician, and tai chi chih instructor. She was trained in China and has worked with the Dalai Lama's personal physician. She has been in practice for thirty years.

An international speaker and workshop leader, Victoria applies the ancient secrets of Eastern medicine to health in the new millennium to reduce stress and revitalize and rejuvenate body, mind, and spirit. She has appeared on Jane Seymour's *Healthy Living* on PBS and has been a featured speaker for Senator John McCain's women's groups. Victoria owns East/West Rejuvenation Oriental Day Spa and Wellness Center in Scottsdale, Arizona. She also works at the Hotel Valley Ho in Scottsdale and in the OH Spa during its Urban

Renewal Retreats, and she certifies people in facial rejuvenation for RainStar University. She holds rejuvenation retreats in Scottsdale and in Hawaii and is available for personal consultations, facial sessions, workshops, and retreats. Currently, she is at work on a companion workbook and workshop for *Ancient Secrets of Facial Rejuvenation*. Her website is www.ewrejuvenationcenter.com, and she invites you to email her at victoria@east-westcenter.com.